The Power of Mental Discipline

The Willpower, Mental Toughness, and Self-Control to

Resist Temptation and Achieve Your Goals

Table of Contents

Introduction

We often tend to perceive discipline negatively or even believe that it is only established in times of crisis or conflict. On the contrary, it depends on all the moments of everyday life including the pleasant moments.

In fact, the word discipline derives its meaning from the word "disciple" which means "teacher-pupil". We can therefore consider discipline as being a teaching coming from the parents and for the child, a training coming from the parents. The goal of discipline is not to make the child "obey" immediately, but to teach him to acquire self-control: that is, self-discipline. It is through the application, on the part of the parents, of a set of rules which tell the child what to and should not do.

The goal of discipline is also to transmit to the child valuesto which he adheres. This therefore leads the child to decide on his own what will be good for him and gradually leads him towards the development of his autonomy, his judgment, his responsibility as well as respect for himself and others.

The hardest thing in the world is knowing how to think. But what does it mean to know how to think? Thinking is a useful activity only if thought turns into action, if it creates something tangible, something to be experienced in the physical world. Here, having mental discipline means being able to control your thinking to make it useful for your existence.

We can think in infinite ways: we can think actively, passively, we can doubt, generate anxiety, fear, restlessness, serenity ... But if you really want to awaken the power of the mind you only need one thing: discipline !

The mind is a muscle and like all muscles it must be trained. Until a few years ago I was a champion ... a champion of self-harm. I was so involved in my mental processes that I had turned into them, I no longer managed anything that was going on in my skull.

Harmful thoughts turned into harmful actions. All the useless that my mind proposed to me generated terrifying moods with consequent paranoid attitudes. Instead of choosing out of love, I chose out of fear. I thought I loved myself but I actually hated myself, I sucked. I was in a negative vortex from which it seemed impossible to get out... but nothing is impossible and everything changes, fortunately. I took a serious risk of not being able to share this piece of life with you

But why did this happen? Because I still did not understand that I was not the mind, I was, I am and will always be outside my thinking : I am the observer and I can choose which thoughts to feed and which to abandon. In every moment I choose who to be and how to be. Every moment we progressed my future experiences.

I will tell you my secret to clear your mind of negative thoughts. When such a thought enters my mind, I visualize it as if it were written on a piece of paper. So I mentally set it on fire and visualize it burning to ashes. Negative thinking is destroyed, and will never enter again - Bruce Lee

Emotions do not generate themselves, we are the creators of them. By controlling our thoughts we are able to manage emotions without the need to repress them. Emotions are the physiological reaction of the thoughts we choose to keep alive, they are the responses to external events that occur and these responses are determined by the (mental) attitude we choose to adopt. And attitude is something that trains over time.

And do you want to know what was the first thing I did that allowed me to regain control of my mind? I stopped listening to her. It's as if for a lifetime you trust someone's advice and inevitably, every time, you find yourself with the c ... o on the ground. After a while, won't you stop listening to him too? And so I did. I let my mind see it for itself and I went out, I went out into the world. I started exercising regularly, I started dedicating myself to the only aspect that brings real change in a person's life: action.

Today I want to share with you some aspects that allowed me to find myself out of the negative mental vortex in which I had slipped.

Even today I know many people who sit on the edge of the bed and think ... and think, think, think. Staring into space, with a finger they scratch their heads and with the mind they are lost in the uselessness of probabilities. High performance anxiety generators, or simply poor souls who cannot extricate themselves from the tangle of their own thoughts. They are the same people who stay in the shower for an

3

hour... and think, think, think. They are the ones you find standing in front of a mirror who worry excessively about their skin, their physical appearance, what other people think and, guess what, they think, think, think....

They are people I love, people for whom, however, I can do nothing but lead by example. And what I would simply like to say is: don't think, you don't need it if you don't know how to do it! Just live!

Here are the 4 steps I followed to discipline the mind and regain control:

1 - STOP THINKING, START TO OBSERVE: is it possible to live without thinking?!? Sure, and how! Observe any animal, identify yourself... and enlighten! Choose to live in the here & now, listen to what happens, be present in your present. In this space-time place unknown to many there is Life. It exists only here and nowhere else your mind chases. Observe the world around you, what happens? Who's that whistling on that branch? And that car that passed was a nice color? Will that child be able to finish the ice cream without dropping it? Is that woman in those 12 heels in pain or is she comfortable? That flower was born only in the middle of the meadow, has anyone seen it? The life that happens outside encourages you to observe it. Looking inside yourself is important, but you have to be able to do it, and looking outside is a great mind-trainer! In the long run you will find that it is very possible to live without thinking. You can also simply choose to live.

2 - MORNING DISCIPLINE: waking up to go to work is already an excellent exercise in discipline, of course. But things that go on for a long time become habit and do not allow us to go beyond our limits, to improve ourselves. Do you want to discipline the mind? Wake up half an hour earlier than usual. Here you will have the proof if you control her or she controls you. If you manage to win that desire that invites you to stay under the covers, you are already halfway there. Spend that half hour on something useful for achieving your goals. 30 minutes a day can change your life!

3 - PHYSICAL DISCIPLINE: mind and body are in close connection with each other and communicate incessantly. Do you want to change your thoughts instantly? Change physiology! Notice: certain thoughts / moods correspond to certain postures. And here if you look around you you can instantly understand who is depressed, who is enthusiastic, who is serene. Just look at his body to get closer to understanding what he is feeling. Do you want to help someone change their mood? Invite him to change physiology! Most of the times it is enough to simply correct your posture to make the miracle happen, to make our mind start to process the information that arrives in a different way. And of course, worrying about doing physical activity every day, of any kind,

4 - CULTURAL DISCIPLINE: choosing what to feed our mind with is essential to give it direction. Everything we feed her is metabolized unconsciously. If you spend your time reading gossip magazines, listening to crime news, taking an interest in someone else's life, what results do you think you will achieve? It's as if you only ate fries, rum and chocolate. What are you waiting for to come out of the intestine?!? The mind gives birth to ideas, nurtures insights and develops according to the quality of the information you choose to offer it. Disciplining the mind also means forcing oneself, forcing oneself to sit down with a book that can help us improve, it means taking pen and paper and writing what we learn from reading. As tiring as it may be at first, this could become one of the most useful and healthy habits you can decide to make yours!

Do you think you have a disciplined mind that does what you want, or an undisciplined mind that goes where it wants?

Imagine having a mind of steel, cold as ice and stepping into the ring completely focused, resistant and persistent in everything without ever losing sight of your goal.

To create a mind of ice you don't have to become a Tibetan monk and lock yourself in a monastery, but you can do it from the comfort of your home.

NO-MIND

A mind centered to the point of blocking negative thoughts until you enter the state called "NO MIND".

The state in which conscious thought is literally blocked, having access to full cognitive behavioral faculties, to one's technical skills with such ease that it becomes a natural process of the mind.

A calm and centered mind that allows you to fight in an intuitive way called a "state of flow".

That state everyone is talking about, the moment in which you make the right move at the right time without even having to think about it, like the classic KO blow.

It just happens without the intervention of the rational part.

Remember that anything that can happen unintentionally can also happen voluntarily if the right tools are used in the right way.

Here are some interesting questions.

Where are you?

What time is it?

What are you?

I guess you would say in the first place: home, kitchen, work, gym, bar etc.

What time is it: You would look at the clock.

What are you? You would start thinking.

Simple questions, simple answers, the difference is how they are evaluated and received.

Here are the correct answers from a present and disciplined mind!

Where are you? Here!

What time is it? Now!

What are you? This moment!

We continually seek information from the outside because we think it is never enough, as if something is always missing.

Once one of my hypnosis masters in a moment that I wanted to know everything immediately told me:

"Stop looking for information from the outside and start looking for it within yourself because that's where you will find the source of your experience."

All this takes discipline and specific training to access your source of knowledge, to your emotional intelligence, your unconscious, entering into the state of flow. Once trained Thy mind in this state will be amazed of the coldness and mental concentration you will have. You will erase all the junk and distractions that distract you from your goal.

Possible?

YES.

What do you need to do?

Train the right way.

Why is this possible?

Because we mainly use the rational mind and not much the unconscious one.

Each works in a completely different way.

WHAT DOES IT MEAN TO ENTER THE STATE OF FLOW?

Entering a state of flow means entering a state of light trance in which the brain waves are low (between Alpha and Theta waves).

Everything happens naturally and the actions and gestures of the subject follow one another according to an internal logic (unconscious process).

It does not seem to be managed by conscious thought, but it is as if someone or something takes over the situation for it to the point of FORGETTING time, judgment and THINKING ITSELF.

No distractions, no useless thoughts, no internal dialogue, just pure action!

Entering the State of Flow means Saying or Doing the right thing at the right time automatically without thinking about it.

See the classic knockout blow, it comes instinctively without thinking about it.

Rational thinking is slow, unconscious thinking is immediate and automatic!

WHAT DOES THIS MEAN?

The rational mind is much slower to process than the emotional one, plus scholars claim that it handles up to 7 pieces of information simultaneously.

The unconscious mind is able to manage a much greater number of them automatically, therefore faster and more responsive.

In short, joining Flow means saying or doing the right thing at the right time without having the idea, becoming PURE ACTION.

Contrary to what happens when the rational part is mainly used.

You know when during an argument with a person you start to hesitate because you don't have the answer ready even if you know what to say?

You have the word on the tip of your tongue, you become hesitant but it doesn't come.

Well, and have you ever done what to when these words come that you were unable to say at that moment?

When it is too late, when the tension has subsided and therefore also the brain waves, the heartbeat and the breath have started to circulate again.

In practice it is as if you had to take a box from a huge shelf in a very short time, and that haste no longer makes you see things where they are even if you have it in front of your eyes.

Vision becomes blurred and emotions take over until you lose the connection with yourself.

WHAT DOES IT MEAN?

It means that we are used to using mainly the logical part of the brain, and less the emotional one because in the gym the emotions are calm.

In the ring, on the other hand, emotions and brain waves are high, and therefore the emotional part comes into play, which if not trained can create problems.

Myths of Mental Discipline

It is one of the most common myths in our culture: Mental Discipline

The myth is bigger than the reality. Benjamin Franklin had them, with his early awakenings, his virtue checklists and his daily reflections. The best athletes have the discipline of training harder than anyone to win gold. My readers often think I am very disciplined when they find out how much I have changed in my life, my new habits and successes which now range from being able to wake up early to being able to save money.

Yet this is all just a myth.

I hope if you accept that this is a myth, you will be relieved of the guilt of not being so disciplined, and you will have the power to create the habits you want without the need for this mythical discipline.

Why discipline is a myth

I wrote about the illusion of discipline before about 4.5 years ago , but it is necessary to revisit the subject from time to time. Especially when I read articles and books that spread this myth. I must therefore put an end to this myth now.

Here's the catch: Discipline seems like a perfectly valid concept, until you dig a little deeper.

Discipline is no mystery.

Except that it is. What is discipline? How disciplined are you? How can you improve your level of discipline? If it's through practice, then how do you train if you don't have it from the start? If you don't feel like doing something, how can you use discipline to force yourself to do it?

I have had many conversations with people who believe deeply in the myth of discipline. This usually happens as follows:

Me : What exactly is discipline? How is this different from motivation (which is the set of actions that we can actually do)?

Friend : Motivation pulls you towards what you want to do, makes you want to do it. Discipline prompts you to do something, makes you do something that you don't want to do.

Me : Ok, so if I don't have discipline, how do I find it?

Friend : You train. It's like a muscle that gets stronger by training it.

Me : And how do I train if I don't have discipline?

Friend : Just do something small, then practice over and over again.

Me : But it takes discipline to do that. What specific action do I need to do to get myself to do something I don't want to do?

Friend : Do you push yourself to do it anyway?

Me : But that requires a discipline that I don't have. Ok, let's say I'm on my couch and I want to go out and run, or get up and write. How do I get this done? What specific action should I take?

Friend : Hmmm! You visualize the end result, the thing you want to do.

Me : But that's a motivational action, not discipline.

Friend : Okay! So plan for rewards. No, it's also motivation. Hmmm. You get in shape and you tell yourself you can do it. No, it's still motivation. You tell people you're gonna do it. Hmm, motivation too. You focus on the positive... or, maybe you just do the things you love to do. But that's still motivational stuff. Uh ...

Every specific action you can take to get yourself to do something is motivation. No discipline.

And that's why discipline is a myth. That might sound good, but it's not a useful concept. When there is a need for specific actions to get you to do something, the only things you can do are motivation. No discipline. I have challenged people to find me motivating discipline action for years now, and no one has succeeded.

Build habits through consistency

When people talk about wanting discipline in their lives, they usually actually want to be more consistent in something. Maybe it is exercise, or meditation, writing, or some other creative activity, or finances, eating, or productivity at work.

All of this is doable without this concept of discipline. What you want is more to build habits.

Habits are not well understood by most people, which is why I created a course (link to his site , in English). In this course, I explore the concept of triggers, positive and negative spirals, consistency, motivation, responsibility, support, and other things that help form habits.

But none of these concepts are nebulous. They are all specific actions you can take to form a habit. If you want to be consistent in something, take the necessary actions to make it a habit. Start small, this way you will be able to build that habit. Once the habit is created (which can take two weeks or several months), you can use it as a basis for further improvement.

Habits are the key to consistency. Not discipline.

And I can attest to that: once you've built a positive, consistent habit, it's a wonderful thing. You feel disciplined, strong and good, even though you experience yourself as the embodiment of this myth.

This is kind of how the Greek gods must have felt.

Mastery In Mental Discipline

A craftsman is master of his craft through repeated practice, with constant care and learning, with devotion towards his goal.

The same goes for mastering the art of discipline:

- A repeated practice
- A resolute devotion to a goal
- Constant learning
- Attention

Approaches

I thought about what was needed to master the art of the mental discipline, and found a few practices that were extremely helpful:

1. **Do your task even when you are not in the mood.** Procrastination is such a common problem that I think it's universal. The main reason we procrastinate, without admitting it personally, is, "I'm not in the mood for this. The task is probably difficult or confusing, and therefore it is uncomfortable, and you would rather do simpler things, which you are good at. You'd rather tidy up the house or do your nails or check your emails instead of starting to write the next chapter of your book. But if we wait until we are in the mood, we will never master life. Instead, practice this:Commit to doing a task, and start doing it, no matter what. Don't let

yourself check email, or social media, or go clean up whatever, or do a chore or a quick errand. Sit down, and do it. It will be uncomfortable. You can still do it, even if it's uncomfortable.

2. **Exercise even when you really don't feel like it.** Yes, it is the same as for procrastination; we delay the exercise for various reasons, usually because it is difficult and we would prefer to do something simpler. But I see it as something I need to do to take care of myself, like eating healthy and brushing my teeth. You wouldn't stop brushing your teeth for a week, would you? Your teeth would rot. Likewise, not exercising for weeks rots your body. Instead, practice this:tell yourself that you are going to be doing a workout / jogging at some point, then get to work. Do this even if you are tired or feeling lazy. Ignore the feeling of laziness, the distraction, clear it from your mind. You will find that you will feel good for doing it. This way, you will begin to master the things that are uncomfortable.

3. **Sit still feeling hungry.** We tend to panic when we are hungry, and rush to the nearest junkyard. What I learned is that you can be hungry and it's not the end of the world. We don't always need to be sated and satisfied with incredibly delicious food. Instead, practice this: don't eat if you're not hungry. When you are hungry, just sit there for a while and turn to the hunger, and see how it feels. It's not that bad. This practice is not meant to starve you (not great), but to show you that a little discomfort won't ruin your life, and that you can make conscious choices about when and how to eat.

4. **Talk to someone about something uncomfortable.** We avoid difficult conversations because they are not funny. They are scary, uncomfortable. But it leads to all kinds of problems, including resentment, a bad relationship, a worsening situation, and more. Instead, practice this:when you have a problem with someone, instead of replaying the problem in your head, talk to the person kindly, with compassion. Try to see the situation from their perspective, not just yours. Bring that up with a simple "Hey, can we talk about ___?" And tell her how you feel, without accusing her or making her feel defensive. Ask her how she feels about it. Approach it with the attitude of finding a solution that works for both of you, that preserves your relationship. What this teaches you is that getting over this awkward situation will solve a lot of difficult problems.

5. **Stick to your habit.** One of the hardest things people face with changing a habit is sticking to that habit after their initial enthusiasm wears off. It's easy to stick to a habit for a week, but what drives you during the second and third week? It gets a lot easier after three weeks, but a lot of people give up the habit too soon. Instead, do this: Commit to a little habit for two months. Do it five minutes a day, and do it at the same time each day, with as many reminders as possible so you don't forget. Record the habit on a calendar or journal, to see your progress. Go there every day and do it. You will begin to master the formation of new habits, which will open up all kinds of changes.

6. **Turn to the problem.** When we have a problem, we often don't even think about it. Ask yourself if you have any of these problems: you avoid exercise, you are overweight, you avoid a major project, you put off managing your finances, you are not happy with a certain situation in your life . Often times these are uncomfortable situations, and we prefer not to face them. Instead, practice this:see the obstacle as the path. Do not avoid the obstacle (the difficult situation, the problem that you are afraid of), do not go around it, do not ignore it. Turn to him. See it. Acknowledge it. Find out what's going on. Find out how to navigate this issue. You'll find it's not easy, but not as bad as you thought it would be, and you'll be glad you did. And more importantly: you will get better at dealing with the problem.

7. **See the good in this activity.** Discipline is really learning that you don't need an incredible reward; there is good in just doing this activity. For example, if you are going to eat balanced meals, you don't need to taste it like your favorite dessert or fried food (reward foods); you can just enjoy the activity of eating fresh and healthy food. If you are going to play sports, you don't need to have a flat stomach or nice arms; you can just enjoy the activity. Practice this: No matter what type of activity, find the good in it, and the activity becomes the reward.

8. **Meditate.** People think meditation is difficult or mystical, but it is quite simple. Practice this: Take 2 minutes to stand still and focus on your breathing, noticing when your mind wanders and gently returning to your breathing. There are other ways to meditate, but this is the easiest, and it shows you how to

observe the urges that emerge and see that you don't need to act and follow those urges.

Strategies

I've always found a way to re-motivate myself and here are some tips I learned that might help:

1. **A goal.** When I am demotivated I have found that it is often because I have too much going on in my life. I try to do too much. And it saps my energy and my motivation. This is probably the most common mistake people can make: They try to do too much, trying to accomplish too many goals at the same time. You cannot maintain your energy and focus (the two most important things in achieving a goal) if you are trying to achieve 2 or more goals at the same time. It is not possible - I have tried many times. You have to pick a goal for now and focus on it completely. I know, it's hard. Nevertheless, I speak from experience. You will still be able to accomplish your other goals when you accomplish your number 1 goal.

2. **Find inspiration.** Inspiration, for me, comes from others who have achieved what I want to achieve, or are in the process of doing it. I read other blogs, books, magazines. I Google my goals, and read success stories. Zen Habits is also a place to be inspired, not just from me but also from many readers who have achieved amazing things.

3. **Get excited.** It may seem obvious, but a lot of people don't think about it much: if you want to re-motivate yourself, make

sure you are excited about your goal. But how do you do this when you don't feel motivated? Well, that starts with inspiration that others can give (see above), but you have to use that excitement and build on it. For me, I learned that by talking to my wife, and others, by reading as much as possible about the subject, and visualizing what it would be like to be successful (seeing the benefits of my goal in my head), I get excited about this goal. Once I do that, the rest becomes just a matter of keeping that energy and nurturing it.

4. **Build anticipation.** This is going to sound harsh, and a lot of people are not going to apply this trick. But it really does work. If you've found inspiration and want to accomplish a goal, don't start right away. Many of us will be excited and want to get started right away. It is a mistake. Plan a date in the future - a week or two, or even a month - and make it your Start date. Mark it on a calendar. Get excited about this date. Make it the most important date of your life. Meanwhile, start writing a plan. And do some of the steps below. Because by delaying your departure, you build anticipation, and you increase your focus and energy for this goal.

5. **Display your goal.** Print your goal in large letters. Build up your goal with a few words, like a mantra ("Sport 15 mins. Daily"), and stick it on your wall or refrigerator. Put it in your home and at your work. Put it on your computer tower. You want to have big reminders about your goal, so you can stay focused and keep your excitement high. A picture of your lens (like a model with a sexy bra, for example) can also help.

6. **Make a public commitment.** No one likes to look silly in front of others. We will go a little further to accomplish something that we have publicly stated. For example, when I wanted to run my first marathon, I started by writing a column about it in my local newspaper. The entire island of Guam(pop. 160,000) knew my goal. I couldn't go back, and even when my motivation dropped, I stuck to my goal and completed it. Now you don't need to commit to your goal at the journal level, but you can do it with friends and family and colleagues, and you can do it in your blog if you have it. a. And be responsible - don't sign up just once, but do it regularly by showing everyone your progress steps every week or so.

7. **Think about it every day.** If you think about your goal every day, there is a much greater chance that it will come true. To this end, displaying your goal on a wall or on your computer (as mentioned above) helps a lot. Sending you daily reminders also helps. And if you can manage to do one little thing to move towards your goal (even just 5 minutes) every day, your goal will almost certainly come true.

8. **Find support.** It's hard to accomplish something on your own. When I decided to run a marathon, I had the help of my friends and family, and I had a large community of runners in Guam who encouraged me to do 8 kilometer runs and who did long endurance races with me. When I decided to quit smoking, I signed up for an online forum and it helped me tremendously. And of course my wife Eva helped me every step of the way. I couldn't have accomplished these goals without her, or without

the others who have supported me. Find your support network, whether in the real world or online, or both.

[ad # zen-milieu-ab]

9. **Realize that there is an ebb and flow.** Motivation is not a constant thing that is always there for you. It comes and it goes, and it comes and goes again, like the wave. But realize that while she can go away, she never does so permanently. She will come back. Hang in there and wait for your motivation to return. Meanwhile, read about your goal (see above), ask for help (see above), and do some of the other things listed here until your motivation returns.

10. **Hang on.** Whatever you do, don't give up. Even if you don't feel motivated today, or this week, don't give up. Once again, motivation will return. Think of your goal as a long trip, and that your pump stroke is just a little junkie in your path. You can't give up on every little addict. Hold on for the long haul, step over the ebb and ride the ebb, and you will get there.

11. **Start small. Really small.** If you see them all in the beginning, it might be because you're thinking too big. If you want to exercise, for example, you may think that you have to do intense sessions 5 days a week. No - take small, tiny, tiny steps instead. Just 2 minutes of exercise. I know, it sounds soft. But it works. Commit to 2 minutes of exercise daily for a week. You might want to do more, but just stick with 2 minutes. It's so easy, you can't fail. Do it at the same time, every day. Just a few

sit-ups, 2 push-ups and a little jogging on the spot. Once you've done this for 2 minutes a day for a week, increase it to 5, and hold for a week. In a month, you will be at 15-20. Want to get up early? Don't think about getting up at 5 a.m. Instead, consider getting up 10 minutes earlier for a week. That's all. Once you've done that, get up 10 earlier again. Small steps.

12. **Build on your little successes.** Again, if you start small for a week, you are going to find success. You can't fail if you start with something ridiculously easy. Who can't exercise for 2 minutes? (If that's you, I'm sorry.) And you'll feel successful, and good about yourself. Use that feeling of success and build on it, with one new small step. Add 2-3 minutes to your exercise routine, for example. With each step (and each step should last at least a week), you will feel even more successful. Take each step really, really small, and you won't fail. After a few months, your small steps will add up to a lot of progress and a lot of success.

13. **Read about it daily.** When I lose my motivation, I just read a book or a blog about my goal. It inspires and invigorates me. For different reasons, reading helps motivate you and keeps you focused on the topic you are reading about. So read about your goal every day, if you can, especially if you don't feel motivated.

14. **Call for help when your motivation drops.** You have problems ? Ask for help. Send me an email. Register on an online forum. Find a partner who will join you. Call your mother. It doesn't matter who, just tell them your problems,

and talking about it will help. Ask them for advice. Ask them to help you overcome this obstacle. It works.

15. **Think about the benefits, not the hardships.** A common problem is that we think about how hard something is. Exercising seems difficult! Just thinking about it tires you out. But instead of thinking about how hard it is, think about what you're going to get out of it, think about how great you'll feel when you're done, and how healthier and leaner you'll be in the long run. The benefits of your goal will help energize you.

16. **Squash negative thoughts; replace them with positive ones.** On top of all of this, it's important to start paying attention to your thoughts. Acknowledge the negative monologues, which is what really causes your demotivation. Just spend a few days being aware of your negative thoughts. Then, after a few days, try squashing them like a bug, and replacing them with a corresponding positive thought. Squash "It's too hard!" and change it to "I can do it! If that Leo weakling can do it, I can do it too! ". It sounds trite, but it works. Really.

Role of Mental Strength

Mental strength is primarily about the correct attitude - but also about maintaining it! Many can build momentum, but constantly motivating yourself is a science in itself.

In order to know what we want to train / improve, we must first define it precisely: Mental strength is a series of character traits or attributes that allow a person to get through a **difficult situation** . A difficult situation is not tied to time in this context, ie it is about short-term mental strength, for example within a workout, and long-term mental strength, for example in a diet or a stressful job. The **mindset** for mental strength combines the following attributes:

- discipline
- motivation
- concentration
- resistance
- Self-confidence
- Determination

2) The **benefits** of trained mental strength are obvious: increased performance, longer stamina and less fear of difficult tasks. This can be transferred to sport, but can also be used in everyday life. Whether it's a tough job, a hobby that requires high concentration or studying for an exam. Because every attribute, for example discipline, can also be improved by training mental strength. The advantages are therefore holistic and diverse.

3) Training **psychology** is different from training your body. It requires different methods and involves different circumstances. But we cannot always control our thoughts either. While trainers and coaches can show us exercises and observe our execution, we rely on ourselves for mental reinforcement.

And now let's get down to business. Here are...

The seven most efficient tips for mental strength:

1. **Take responsibility** . The first step in training and building up mental strength is taking responsibility. For everything in life. We like to make ourselves comfortable, because humans are naturally lazy animals. He seeks an **excuse** for everything bad that happens to him in life: "I'm fat because I have bad genes". "I'm just lazy, that's how it is." "I can't do it because X ...". Everyone knows the game, because everyone has already looked for an excuse for something that makes it easier for them. Because it removes responsibility. But when everything in life is faced and takes responsibility for every circumstance and every action, one is also more satisfied with what one achieves. **satisfaction**is an important asset in life and to be able to write **success** and thus satisfaction on your shoulder feels very good. That motivates and makes you hungry for more.

The automatic result is that you leave nothing to chance and thus forge your own happiness. Because what you control, you can control. **To Do** : start taking responsibility for everything in your life !

2. **Create awareness**. The next step is to create awareness of strengths and weaknesses, advantages and disadvantages, good and bad. Because not being aware of something bad causes **insecurity** , which in turn leads to mental weakness. If you know what you're bad at, you can work on it. But "creating awareness" also includes accepting weaknesses . By the way, none of them are free, everyone has weaknesses. There is an Achilles tendon for everyone and everything. If you manage to recognize and accept weaknesses, you can work on them and turn them into strengths. This is the next path to mental strength . **To Do** : Make yourself aware of your weaknesses and strengths !

3. Using **momentum.** Some things or events give us a tremendous boost. For example, take a look at the video below and you will feel an incredible amount of motivation. Often, however, this momentum is only enough for a short time. It is important to understand that moment bored short and you from the power of 1 angfristige motivation must draw. Let's take the typical good resolutions at the beginning of the year as an example: "I want to lose weight" or "I want to quit smoking". After 2 weeks of motivation, everything is forgotten. This lack of mental strength is related to the fact that many are **unaware of** the momentumare. If you understand that you are

27

likely to be motivated at the beginning, but dry spells and also tougher times (= resistance) will come, you can be prepared for this and will not be thrown directly off track when they occur. **To Do** : Use momentum and be aware that it is disappearing !

4. **Think positive**. The next step is to **constantly** think **positively**. It's a little difficult at first, but mental strength doesn't come from pessimism. To gloss over everything inside is not the goal, but always to start with the **best result** . In this way, one fades out negative and thus braking thoughts and concentrates on success. **To Do:** Always think positively and assume the best !

5. **Use visualization.** Next, it is important that you always visualize positively. As a result, you automatically concentrate on the upcoming and ignore the unimportant. With positive thinking, positive visualization is the most difficult quality of mental strength. Because sometimes the task ahead is difficult and seems unrealistic to master. However, precisely because of this, one must practice, practice, practice these two qualities . Regardless of whether it is about the result of a decision, whether you lift a heavy weight or run a marathon and prepare yourself for it internally: (**To Do**) visualize the process and the positive result!

6. **Set goals**. If you keep setting yourself new goals, you will continue to develop. Standing still is death, both for every living being and for every society or company. Through constant further development and striving for higher / new goals, you consolidate your mental strength. In the end, you

will reach a level that you would not have believed yourself capable of and that makes you mentally strong and motivates you. **To Do**: Set yourself small and large goals again and again so that you can constantly develop yourself!

7. **Music**. Musk is a fantastic way to motivate yourself again and again.If you listen to motivating music before a difficult task or a hard workout, you are automatically more productive: your thoughts adjust to the stress, you remember your goals and the reasons for which you set yourself the task and you can focus on it focus the workout. **To Do**: Find music that motivates you and listen to it before every workout / task !

8. **Bonus: discipline**. The last point is about practicing discipline, because it is an incredible driver for motivation, hardness and thus **mental strength**. Discipline is not easy, everyone gets weak. But don't let that discourage you, instead face the discipline over and over again. Discipline includes **resilience** and **control** . The following three tasks will train your discipline tremendously and at the same time show you how resilient you can actually be! There is nothing bigger in any of the three tasks. Neither will kill you nor harm you. It's all in the head!

To Do 1 : Eat 10 raisins in 10 minutes.

To Do 2 : Just skip dinner.

To Do 3 : Sit on the floor for 10 minutes and try not to think about anything. Set a timer or a clock to exactly 10 minutes.

These tips and exercises will help you understand what mental strength is and how to train it.

How does mental training work?

In mental training or mental coaching, resilience, motivation and discipline are trained. Mental training is not the same as motivational training or MAT (mental activation training). Mental training is more about athletic performance and the optimization of movement sequences. Common methods of behavior therapy are applied to exercise physiology and the following aspects are addressed:

- Forecast training
- Attention regulation
- Self-talk regulation

The actual execution should be improved through the intensive presentation of the sequence of movements, as one can feel the process internally and empathize with the movement.

Prepared by tensing and relaxing. You first tense the muscles specifically for a few seconds and then loosen them again. This also has the advantage of focusing on the muscles that will be most stressed in the following movement / exercise. This is exactly what bodybuilders do when they are actively focused on the muscle they are training in the gym.

Attention regulation is especially useful if you find it difficult to concentrate. The aim here is to direct the perception specifically to the upcoming event. The concentrated concentration means that the mental aspect of the exercise is 100% guaranteed and the performance from then on depends on the physical condition.

With the help of prognosis training you can practice setting your expectations correctly. Through the improved assessment of the result or the specific target expectation, you can better adjust to performance and gain confidence in your abilities. This in turn leads to increased self-confidence .

Self-Discipline & Its Development

Self-discipline can be defined as the outward manifestation of your inner strength. Thanks to it, you make deliberate choices. You are no longer driven by your bad habits, emotions, circumstances or the influence of others. It is an essential skill for self-improvement , but also one of the most difficult to master and to implement. To develop it, two things are needed: cultivating qualities like enthusiasm, tenacity, courage and optimism, and taking concrete steps to take action.

A self-disciplined person evolves in a stimulating environment, acts consistently over a period of time, is willing to take risks , sees his self-esteem increase , influences the lives of those around him, and continues to move forward to achieve his goals. Goals.

1. Identify your obstacles and your motivations

It's all about doing some soul-searching to figure out what's stopping you from being more disciplined. It is important to identify the blocking factors in order to know how to transform them.

Why do you need more discipline? What are your motivations? Your sources of inspiration? Developing self-discipline requires having a strong desire to achieve a specific goal. Otherwise, you'll have a hard time staying focused for long periods of time. Ask yourself, "What do I want? "," Why do I want it? "," Why do I have to do this? "

2. Define what you want

Self-discipline can only last if it is directed towards something specific. This outcome could be a goal you want to achieve, a habit you want to develop, or a behavior you want to change. So you need to be very clear about what you want to achieve . This thing must be close to your heart. It's your fuel, what gets you up in the morning. This lens should be powerful enough to get you through the toughest times.

In general, most people frame their goals around the 4 areas that have the most influence on your life: health, family, money, and themselves.

The health is related to your well-being, your body, your ability to live your life. The family about your immediate surroundings, the people around you that are the basis on which you have an impact on the world. The money is the tool that allows you to reorder the world according to your expectations. And the person refers to the notions of growth and learning, and how you see the world.

Once the goal is identified, determine the habits and behaviors that will help you achieve the desired result. In other words, what kind of person do you need to be in order to reach your goal? What you do should reflect your core values. This is the only way to ensure that your long term goal is met.

3. Set SMART goals

Your goal should be:

- Specific: Make sure the goal is specific. Don't just say "exercise then work". Instead, say "Stretch for 30 minutes and then finish my lesson for English class." Don't make a goal complex. The simpler it is, the more chances you have of achieving it.

- Measurable: Make sure you can measure progress in quality or quantity. For example, avoid an objective like "write the first part of a new article". Instead, favor something like "write 500 words of a new article".

- Achievable: Be able to achieve your goal. Don't plan to work 16 hours a day for a month, you won't be able to. In any case, not in a healthy and efficient way. Ambition is essential in achieving a goal, but it must be accessible.

- Realistic: Avoid getting into things that are very unlikely to happen. Pick a relevant and realistic goal that is ambitious enough to be a challenge, but that is within your skills. Otherwise it will become a source of anxiety and you will give up.

- Temporarily defined : Delimit the objective in time with a beginning and an end otherwise you will never end. If you haven't reached your goal by your planned end date, there's nothing stopping you from setting a new one. But it is important to set limits.

4. Find suitable models

It's a long road, and it's easy to feel lonely on this trek, but rest assured you're not the first person on it. Many others have been there before you. After thinking about the goals, identify role models (friends, family, and colleagues) who can inspire you or help you achieve them. These are people who are doing this job right now or who have successfully achieved their goals. Who can you learn from to move forward more effectively?

Take the time to ask these people how they acquired their self-discipline. Ask them what specific actions they took to achieve the desired result. Then, take advantage of their experience, it is a precious help to support you in your work.

Get inspired by models, read about them - biographies are a valuable source of information - watch their interviews, hear their stories. If they did, it means it's possible. So you too can reach the destination.

5. Develop an action plan

Put in place a practical plan of action to help you reach your goal. Break down your goal into more manageable steps. This technique helps you control the tasks you are working on without getting overwhelmed or procrastinating.

As defined in SMART Goals, having a specific deadline helps you discipline yourself, as it focuses your mind on a specific end date for achieving your goal. With this ultimatum in mind, all of your resources and energy are channeled in an appropriate manner to maintain the momentum necessary to carry out your actions. Plus, a deadline gives a sense of urgency, which will help you stay focused and disciplined on the tasks at hand.

6. Set the priority of your tasks and activities

The goal you have chosen is supposed to change your life. Making it a priority is the most important thing you can do right now. Before you do anything, be sure to take the steps to achieve your goal first . Everything else is secondary. In self-discipline, priorities are paramount because they help give your day the structure you need.

When you prioritize effectively, you no longer wonder what needs to be done. Instead, you already know what's most important, and how to structure your day. The more structured you are, the fewer decisions you have to make . With fewer choices, you're less likely to get distracted by irrelevant tasks and activities.

7. Track your progress

Self-discipline flourishes when it is possible to measure progress towards achieving a goal. In this context, it is essential to put in place a process to monitor the progress of your actions . Use a calendar or journal to record your progress. Tracking your results and effectively measuring the progress you are making helps you stay motivated and focused on the tasks at hand.

If you're struggling to hit the milestones you've set for yourself, tracking your progress can help you make any necessary adjustments to stay on track. Watch your results and any temptations that arise. Once identified, make any necessary adjustments to avoid them.

Remember that rarely, if ever, things turn out ideally. There are always unforeseen events. It is part of the process of change. However, with self-discipline, you will be successful in overcoming these obstacles.

8. Engage in a sport activity

Sport is a great way to improve your personal discipline . In addition, physical activity greatly contributes to improving your mental well-being. Participating in physical activity gives you the opportunity to learn how to do your best and to surpass yourself. Then you will integrate this process into your daily life.

9. Forget about excuses and complaints

Making excuses or complaining rarely, if ever, helps to improve a situation. On the contrary, it can even make matters worse.

Problems always happen when you least expect them. But a problem is only your opinion of the situation. Things might be a little different from what you imagine. You just need a change of perspective .

Leaving yourself to hasty conclusions will only sabotage your efforts. Instead, use your imagination constructively to refocus your efforts on what you need to do. If you don't take control of your imagination, you create space for anger or frustration and then apologies and complaints. These may make you feel better, in the very short term, but in no way do they provide a way to overcome the situation.

Stay in control of your emotions to refocus your efforts on what needs to be done to help you reach your goal.

10. Don't wait until tomorrow

How many times have you heard a friend say "I quit smoking next week"? We like to convince ourselves that tomorrow will be easier than today. That we will be better disposed, fitter, more motivated, etc. The reality is different. Tomorrow is rarely better than now .

Postponing, procrastinating, only takes you further away from your goals every day. The best time to start something was yesterday. The second is today .

Say your goal is to save. Where would you be if you started 6 months or 5 years ago? Don't wait until tomorrow. Start now, this is the only valid option.

11. Regulate your emotions

We all know situations where our emotions bring out the worst in us and destroy our self-discipline. Thoughts, emotions and behaviors are intertwined and influence each other . Therefore, when it comes to developing personal discipline and taking action, knowing how to regulate your emotions is very important. Mindfulness is a great tool to help us take control of our emotions and therefore our behavior.

By practicing mindfulness techniques such as meditation, we learn to be aware of our changing emotional states . In doing so, the more attentive we are, the easier it is to notice changes in our emotional states. This technique, combined with acceptance and non-judgment , gives us the ability to stay in touch with our emotions without letting them overwhelm us.

Asceticism & Self-Discipline

Asceticism comes from the Greek word askésis which is originally part of the sports vocabulary and which designates the demanding lifestyle adopted by athletes: diet, sleep, exercises ...

Asceticism implies renouncements, privations. It is a discipline of life. It is a question of imposing a discipline (self-discipline) and thus of exercising one's will against natural tendencies of the body or the mind. Meditation and fasting are thus ascetic practices.

This exercise of the will and this discipline of life remain most of the time in measure and in balance. There are more extreme ascetic practices with the practice of mortifications and penances.

Benefits

Self-discipline is the ability to resist impulses in order to achieve one's goals.

Many American psychologists and coaches have written that self-discipline makes you happy.

Self-discipline and taking charge of yourself would allow you to experience more positive emotions and to be generally more satisfied with your life.

Self-discipline allows you to give up habits that make you unhappy (eating too much sugar, going to bed too late ...).

Also, being able to delay meeting some of your needs just to achieve certain goals leads to a real sense of self-control and that makes you happy!

How to develop more self-discipline?

The will works like a muscle. Self-discipline can therefore develop like a muscle. With practice, it becomes easier to resist impulses.

Developing new habits (food, activity, method) to achieve goals is the essence of self-discipline. Automating new behavior takes a little over two months. Once it is almost automatic, you no longer need

To motivate yourself, think about the advantages of your new inhabitants, not the constraints!

Meditation for more self-discipline

Meditation increases willpower. This has been proven by science. A study carried out by an Italian neuroscientist, for example, showed that people who meditated regularly for 8 weeks had strengthened the part of their brain responsible for self-control.

So to resist impulses more easily, meditate!

For example, you can practice a simple meditation exercise, mindful breathing.

Make yourself comfortable, with your hands on your thighs, eyes open or closed.

Concentrate only on your breathing. Be aware of the movement of your chest and stomach as you breathe, as well as the air coming in and out of your nostrils. When your thoughts drift, slowly regain awareness of your breathing.

Start with a 1 minute exercise to begin with, then gradually move to a 2 or 3 minute exercise.

Overcoming Imposter Syndrome

Have you ever felt like you didn't deserve your place and sooner or later your family, friends or coworkers would notice? That feeling that you were there by chance and that this luck could not last? That someone would eventually unmask you? This feeling is common in many people, it is called "impostor syndrome".

What is impostor syndrome?

A large number of well-known people in their field share an ugly secret: despite their obvious success, they feel illegitimate and attribute their success to luck. For them, this psychological phenomenon reflects the belief that they are incompetent despite objective evidence of success. This lingering feeling that their role should have been given to others drives them to engage in unbridled perfectionism. This heightens their fear of failure and generates anxiety and helps to create a state of depression .

First identified in the 1970s by psychologists Suzanne Imes and Pauline Rose Clance, impostor syndrome was first observed in women and then extended to both sexes. This phenomenon affects nearly 70% of the working population, and applies to successful people, unable to internalize and accept their success . Most of the time, they attribute their accomplishments to luck rather than their qualifications, and fear that others will end up revealing their sham.

This syndrome (which, despite its name, is not a pathology) is often seen as an individual concern and only exists in the minds of those who experience it . We can admire a person for their achievement and imagine them confident and comfortable with their own accomplishments. Even if, inside, it is often only a mass of anxieties, self-criticisms and ruthless judgments towards itself.

When impostors achieve some form of success, they attribute it to others. Thus, they create and maintain the belief of their deception.

The irony of this syndrome is that it is prevalent among the best performing people, that is, those who, logically, are the least likely to experience it. Moreover, when they assess their efforts, accomplishments, and successes logically and without emotion, they can clearly (reluctantly) view them as their own. But they just can't bring themselves to accept it. To consider and to accept are two very different things.

There are a lot of people who think I am an expert. How can they believe this about me? I know so much about everything I don't know. (Margaret Chan - Director General of the World Health Organization between 2007 and 2017)

Success at all costs

According to Suzanne Imes, many people who see themselves as impostors grew up in families that place great importance on success . In particular, when parents send mixed messages, alternating praise and criticism. Then the social pressure only adds another layer to the problem.

Sometimes childhood memories, such as feeling that your grades are never good enough for your parents or that your siblings have outperformed you in certain areas, can have a lasting impact. People often incorporate the idea that to be loved or to be lovable, you have to perform well and achieve a goal.

Factors external to a person, such as the environment, can also play a major role in stimulating a feeling of deception. The more you are surrounded by people who are like you, the more you will feel confident. And conversely, the fewer people there are like you, the greater the negative impact on self-confidence.

The 5 types of impostor

Valerie Young, author of The Secret Thoughts of Successful Women, and an expert on the subject, identified 5 subgroups:

1. The perfectionist
2. Superman / Superwoman
3. The natural genius
4. The individualist
5. The expert

1. The perfectionist

The impostor phenomenon and perfectionism often go hand in hand. So-called impostors believe that every task at hand should be done perfectly, and rarely ask for help. This perfectionism can lead to two typical responses: either procrastinating, or delaying a task for fear of not being able to complete it to the highest standards, or spending more time than necessary preparing and completing the task.

Perfectionists have extremely high expectations, and view a 99% goal as a failure. Any mistake, no matter how small, makes them question their own competence.

For them, success is rarely satisfying, because they always think they can do better. But it is neither productive nor healthy. Recognizing and owning your accomplishments is essential for avoiding burnout, finding contentment, and cultivating self-confidence.

To thwart this type of impostor syndrome, learn to control your mistakes by seeing them as a natural part of the process. Push yourself to take action rather than waiting to be ready . Force yourself to start the project you've been planning for months. The truth is, there will never be a perfect time and your work will never be 100% perfect. The sooner you are able to accept this, the better off you will be.

2. Superman / Superwoman

Supermen / superwomen work harder than those around them to prove that they are not impostors. They feel the need to be successful in all aspects of life - work, family, relationship - and may feel stressed when they don't accomplish something.

This overload of work only covers their insecurity and can harm not only their mental health, but also their relationships with others.

Impostor workaholics are in fact dependent on the validation that comes from the work, not the work itself . It is therefore a matter of getting rid of external validation and of taking constructive criticism rationally, and not personally.

3. Natural genius

When the natural genius has to struggle or work hard to accomplish something, he thinks that means he is not good enough. He's used to quick and easy skills, and when he has to strain, his brain tells him he's proof of his sham.

People in this situation judge success based on their ability and effort. In other words, if they have to work hard for something, they assume they must be bad at it.

These types of impostors set their inner bar at an incredibly high standard, just like perfectionists. But natural geniuses don't just judge themselves based on ludicrous expectations, they also judge themselves by striving to get it right the first time. When they are not able to do something quickly or fluently, their alarm sounds.

To overcome this, you have to see yourself as a work in progress. To accomplish great things, you have to learn throughout your life and develop your skills. Rather than fighting when you don't meet very high standards, you need to identify specific and modifiable behaviors to improve over time.

4. The individualist

Individualists feel that they have to perform tasks themselves and, if they need to ask for help, think that this means that they are incompetent, and therefore impostors. It's fine to be independent, but not if you refuse assistance in order to prove your worth.

5. The expert

Experts feel the need to master every piece of information before starting a project and are constantly looking for new certifications or training to improve their skills. They will not apply for a job if they do not meet all the criteria of the offer. They may be hesitant to ask a question or speak up in a meeting because they are afraid of appearing stupid.

Wanting to boost your skills can certainly help you advance professionally and stay competitive in the job market. But this tendency to constantly seek more information can actually be a form of procrastination. It is then advisable to acquire a skill when it is necessary rather than to store up others for a hypothetical future.

How to treat impostor syndrome?

One of the first steps in overcoming feelings of impostor is to recognize the thoughts and put them into perspective. Simply observing that feeling rather than mobilizing it can be helpful.

You can also reframe your thoughts. The only difference between someone with impostor syndrome and another is the way they respond to challenges. People who do not feel like impostors are neither smarter, nor more competent, nor more capable. This means learning to think like non-impostors and to value constructive criticism.

It is also helpful to share how you are feeling with friends or people you trust. Those with more experience can reassure you that what you are feeling is normal. Knowing that others have been in your shoes can make it seem less scary.

Realize that there is no shame in asking for help when you need it. If you don't know how to resolve a problem, seek advice from a loved one or a therapist.

It's common for people with impostor syndrome to turn down career opportunities because they feel like they're not doing a good job. However, it is important to distinguish between the voice in your head that says you are not competent and the one that rationally recognizes that it is not possible. Remember that exciting new work can open many doors for you. Don't let your inner impostor turn down these game-changing opportunities. These opportunities can help you learn, develop, and advance your career.

Keep in mind Richard Branson's famous line: "If someone offers you an incredible opportunity and you're not sure you can do it, say yes. Then learn how to do it. "

Quotes To End Inner Chaos

1. What troubles men is not things, it is their opinions of them.

2. Don't wait for events to happen as you want them to; decide to want what happens and you will be happy.

3. It doesn't depend on you to be rich, but it depends on you to be happy.

4. It is the mark of a small mind to take it out on another when it fails in what it has undertaken; he who exercises spiritual work on himself will blame himself; whoever completes this work will not blame him or others.

5. No one will harm you unless you agree to it; evil will come only when you judge that you are being harmed.

6. Our salvation and our loss are within ourselves.

7. Make perfect what is in our hands, and take other things as they come.

8. Knowing how to listen is an art.

9. Happiness does not consist in acquiring and enjoying, but in desiring nothing, for it consists in being free.

10. It is wise to accuse only oneself of one's misfortunes.

11. Don't you know that the source of all human miseries is not death, but fear of death?

12. When someone makes you angry, know that it is your judgment that makes you angry.

13. The occasions are indifferent, the use made of them is not.

14. First tell yourself who you want to be, then do what you need to do accordingly.

15. He is a wise man who does not regret what he does not have but rejoices in what he has.

16. He who progresses does not blame anybody, does not praise anybody, does not criticize anybody, does not incriminate anyone. He said nothing, neither of his importance, nor of his knowledge.

17. For me there are only happy omens; because, whatever happens, it depends on me to get some good from it.

18. Freedom is independence of thought.

19. Let us seek our possessions ourselves, otherwise we will not find them.

20. Be silent more often, say only what is necessary and in a few words.

21. Everything is change, not to no longer be but to become what is not yet.

22. It is not through the satisfaction of desire that freedom is obtained, but through the destruction of desire.

23. There is only one road to happiness and that is to give up things that are beyond our control.

The Power Of Gratitude

The world is perfect as it is. Yes, you got it right. There is nothing wrong with what happens. The imperfection is in the point of view that we choose to adopt and which makes us judge whether something is right or wrong. Justice is a trap of the mind , as well as the continuous search for perfection in a reality where everything is already perfect. Don't you think so? Read on please... what happens is just what happens, you can accept it or not, but things don't change. If anything, what changes is you and I assure you that once you have changed yourself, you will have changed everything. Change your image of yourself, change who you are through the power of gratitude, through acceptance, forgiveness and service, and your whole life will change.

The power of gratitude is expressed through a conscious attitude, aware that everything is perfect as it is. If you could not accept this how would you be grateful indiscriminately and unconditionally for this Life that has been granted to you?!? If you can find things that don't go the way they should (in your view), how can you be fully grateful?!?

Let's repeat it: what happens is only what happens and it is neither right nor wrong, but you see the reflection of who you are in the world and based on how you feel you make a judgment.

We don't see things as they are, we see them as we are.
(Anais Nin)

Do you know why we can say that everything is perfect as it is? Because the outside world is a reflection of our inner world. The individual unconscious manifests the individual reality, the collective unconscious manifests the collective reality. This is how the unconscious works. If we all focused on war, the world would fall into chaos, vice versa if we focus on generosity and brotherhood we will return to enjoy the earthly paradise. But even these would continue to be just points of view. Heaven for someone could be hell for someone else ...

You create and manifest realities in line with the mental-emotional images that you let the subconscious absorb and luckily not all of us watch the news, but that's another story ...

If everything manifest is the projection of the manifest, understand that everything you can experience is perfect because it is nothing more than a photocopy of what already exists on a spiritual level within each of us. Everything is the fruit of Love, the universal energy that is eternal in a continuous coming and going between the world of the visible and the invisible.

In nature, nothing is perfect and everything is perfect. Trees can be twisted, bizarrely curved, but still beautiful.

(Alice Walker)

Do you want to change the physical reality? Change the inner reality , this is the only way, the only method that most personal growth gurus avoid telling you. Maybe they don't know it, maybe they know it but they don't want to tell you, maybe they know it but they understand very well that this truth is hard to accept and by promoting it they could lose consensus. But this blog follows the rule of few but good (even if by now few are no longer with my great pleasure and gratitude) , so we don't care and go on, do you agree?

If some things are uncomfortable to accept, perhaps they are also those that come closest to reality, don't you think?!? When an idea is accepted and shared by everyone there is something wrong, you have stopped thinking for yourself.

The rebellious ideas, the ones that make the difference, are those that cause a stir, ignite the fires of the inquisition, but they are also those that allow differentiation, growth and evolution. Sometimes to dare is simply to allow yourself to think differently from the crowd ... sometimes to dare is to simply go back to living in harmony with who we really are, away from stereotypes and prepackaged dogmas useful only to keep the most powerful weapon that exists at bay: your mind!

Now I see the secret to creating the best people. It is growing in the fresh air and eating and sleeping with the earth. (Walt Whitman)

GRATITUDE IS LOVE

AND LOVE IS EVERYWHERE

Everything is perfect as it is, yes, I tell you again. And it is perfect because everything springs from universal energy, from Love, from the One. Love, God, Mother Nature, Jehovah, Tao (no matter what you want to call what unites us and unites us) ... it has no personality, it is not outside you, it is not inside you, it is everywhere, it does not punish and it does not reward, it simply creates, creates what we ask for and wants nothing more for us than what we want for ourselves.

A little twisted? Wait I'll try again: God wants for you what you want for you, better this way?

God has given us a very simple means to communicate with him, to expose our requests. This means are the emotions, or rather, the deep sensations of our soul. When you feel love ask for love and you will receive love, when you feel fear ask for fear and you will receive fear, when you feel gratitude ask for experiences to be even more grateful and these will be attracted to you, to who you are, to how you are.

If with your mind you continue to relive unpleasant episodes in your life, if you continue to feel fear, if you lack confidence in your abilities, if you feel contempt for those who are different from you ... what do you think you will collect tomorrow?

Ask and you shall receive! Tomorrow you will reap what you sow today with your emotional intention, this is what you need to know to create the life you want and to improve the world. Now that you are aware of this, any excuse is void. Every expressed complaint manifests itself in experiences to complain about, every gesture of love expands, infecting every future event. If you want to have more, you must be more, you must be grateful, and then your existence will become filled with every possible joy.

But let's take it one step at a time: why is gratitude so important?

Gratitude is the feeling that comes closest to our true essence, to the Love from which we were originated and of which we are made. The Love that flows in you is the same that flows in an oak. But while for the oak it does nothing but realize the essence that was contained within its acorn, for you it realizes what you continually sow through the power of choice, intention, free will. You choose what to think, Love will only allow the manifestation of your thought in its physical correspondent.

Love is energy that makes you grow, it is energy that manifests the essence of things by realizing itself in perfect harmony with all the information it receives.

Recognizing Love everywhere is the first step in understanding that everything is perfect as it is. Yes, even someone's death is perfect because if it happened it is only because Love has allowed it.

I repeat to you: there are no bad or beautiful things, it is we who make sense of things and we usually define as ugly everything that we do not understand. Just as water from solid becomes liquid, evaporates, condenses and then rains again, so your soul, your essence, before dwelling in your body was elsewhere and so it will be when your body ceases to function. Change is perfection at work! The term death indicates an event that it is not yet possible for us to fully understand because we have not lived it but if Life allows it it means that it is perfect as it is.

What's wrong with death? What are we so mortally afraid of? Why not treat death with a little humanity and dignity and decency and, *God forbid, even humor? Gentlemen, the real enemy is not death. Do we want to fight diseases? Let's fight the most terrible of all: indifference*

(Patch Adams)

RECOGNIZING LOVE GENERATES GRATITUDE

Maybe the preamble I gave you was long but (I hope) it helped to make you understand that there is nothing wrong with everything that happens, really! Perceiving Love everywhere presupposes that it also resides in you, you are the One in the All and at the same time you are All in the One.

God is an infinite sphere, the center of which is everywhere and the circumference nowhere.

(Lao Tzu)

It is your perception that makes you move away from this truth, it is your senses, but when you return to who you really are, you return to the now, every doubt disappears, every problem dissolves because there is no problem, and every fear is shattered because there is only Love. Sometimes you understand it, sometimes you don't...

The only obstacle we have ever had is ourselves and, at the same time, we ourselves are the solution. When you move away from yourself you are creating resistance in the perception of this Truth, that all is Love and is perfect as it is; when you come back to yourself you come back aware and break down any kind of disturbance that interfered with your attunement to the Truth.

The Universe is a balance, nature is a balance, you are a balance. If a certain type of energy becomes unbalanced on one side, its opposite will intensify to counterbalance it and restore balance to the center. Action, reaction. When the energies are balanced, the center appears, when the center appears there is harmony.

If wars, murders, pestilences occur somewhere, it means that peace, generosity and super health are manifested elsewhere ... everything is in balance, the Whole is ONE balance! If it's day here, it's night somewhere else...

Someone has defined the disease of man today as a progressive loss of the center. At one time man was believed to be the measure of all things, later he continued to be believed to be the measure of all things, today he is no longer believed to be the measure of anything.

(Eugenio Montale)

In summary: total acceptance of what is, making aware in the present moment without any kind of resistance, is the origin of true gratitude!

THE POWER OF GRATITUDE:

ACCEPTANCE, FORGIVENESS AND SERVICE

Being truly grateful means understanding that there are no right or wrong things but, simply, things are as they are, period.

Here are the three key steps to tap into your full potential as an intentional creator, a creator who can harness the power of gratitude to improve himself, his life and the world!

ACCEPTANCE

Accepting something does not mean justifying it. If you come across someone's rudeness you can accept their inability to be better than that at the moment but you don't have to justify it, rather feel sorry for them. Instead of being annoyed accept the fact that Love is experiencing itself also through the rudeness of this individual to understand himself and to make you understand something. Accepting what apparently you find unfair leads you to change the perception you have of the event, therefore by changing your feeling, you also change your vibrational offer. By changing what you sow, you change your crop. War is won with peace ...

THE FORGIVENESS

Always staying on the same example, we can also say that reacting to the event in a different way from what you would expect, the event itself will change its course. Accepting leads us to forgive, not to justify, and if you can forgive the rudeness of others, it means that you are bringing light to both the event and the person involved. This is a great opportunity because by doing so, the energies at play are freed up and rudeness (and the individual) is allowed to become aware of itself, therefore to evolve. Forgiveness releases tension and transmutes pain energy into awareness energyfor both parties. Forgiveness does not mean neither denying nor canceling pain, nor being submissive, it means turning what happens into understanding. When we give a higher sense to things than what appears on the surface, it becomes easier for us to see the harmony and perfection of the Whole and the One.

SERVICE

When you take care of Life, Life takes care of you! For this third point, I bring you a reflection that I found on the web and that struck me a lot. I think there is nothing more to add to these words: Rivers do not drink their own water, trees do not eat their fruit, the sun does not shine for itself and flowers do not disperse their fragrance for themselves. Living for others is a rule of nature; life is beautiful when you are happy, but life is extraordinary when others are happy because of you. Our true nature is to be of service to make everything better. Those who do not live to serve do not need to live. Always keep this third point in mind because your whole future is contained here. The service you offer to the Universe, to Life, is the origin of your success as a human being. Be grateful for the opportunity you have to make everything better and work hard to make it so.

If you help others, you will be helped. Maybe tomorrow, maybe a hundred years from now, but you will be helped. Nature has to pay the debt. It is a mathematical law and all life is mathematics.

(George Ivanovitch Gurdjieff)

Bottom Line: Gratitude is the beginning of your happiness, and happiness breeds successful people. When you are grateful, you can't be sad, angry or anxious at the same time, it's impossible. Two different types of frequencies cannot coexist in your body and mind. When you are grateful you shine, when you shine you illuminate, and we know it very well, only light allows things to grow. The inner solution always allows the outer solution to manifest. The way out is inside!

Emotions Management & Mental Discipline

If you were in the middle of a rock concert, right under the stage, and about fifty meters away someone called you, do you think you would hear it? If you were a butterfly and you found yourself in the middle of a storm, would you be able to stay firm on the ground? What if during the concert everything was silenced except the voice that was calling you? What if I get heavy as a tonne boulder in a storm? Things would change drastically right? You would live in a completely different situation. Learning to manage emotions means being able to take the best shape in relation to what is happening, it allows you to change the perception of the world, and meditation and concentration are excellent allies to do so.

We are human beings, we are emotional beings and it is not possible for us to live without generating emotions. But it is one thing to recognize emotions and manage them, it is another thing to be overwhelmed by them. If a driver passes you on the right, honking your horn and gesturing, what reaction would you have?

You could ignore it by returning to focus on the road, or you could inveigh in turn by engaging in a punitive chase, or again, you could give him way because you imagine that he is in a hurry for some emergency, I know, maybe he has to go to the hospital that is being born his son...

What happened in any case does not change: the driver overtook you on the right (the highway code prohibits it), he trumpeted you and gestured something. This is the only certain truth there is, also called objective truth. Your internal reaction will instead determine your reality, the subjective truth. And every reaction you choose will be followed by a certain type of emotion. Yes, you are deliberately choosing what to feel, what to think, therefore what subjective reality to live.

This example reminds us that we interface with the outside world as we are and think and certainly not as things are. Things happen because they have to happen, the world is perfect as it is , you react as you choose to react, so you create the quality of reality in which to move.

Learning to manage your emotions means learning to manage events and not to be overwhelmed by them. It also means learning to manage people and relationships. Everything is connected.

People are emotions that walk. You are a living emotional center. When we relate to others, it is not only the thoughts of individuals that meet and create a confrontation, but also emotions. Training the mind and heart to dialogue allows us to make the most of our potential as human beings, it allows us to receive and offer the best during the time we are allowed to live.

You cannot think that you are making the best of a situation if you are unable to make the best of yourself. Roots create fruits... you can't change fruits if you don't change roots. The only way to get different results is to change yourself.

MANAGING EMOTIONS TO STAY FAITHFUL TO THE GOAL

Unwelcome things happen to everyone in life. Overcoming obstacles is part of our evolutionary process. If we hadn't had difficulty growing up now we wouldn't be who we are, right? And do you know why you managed to be transformed by the difficulties you encountered on your path? Because you had what you wanted in your mind, that's the truth. You have been faithful to the goal you wanted to reach, you have been a rock in the storm, you have not let yourself be beaten down, you have not been stopped. You wanted to learn to walk and hit your butt on the ground until you made it. You wanted to learn to drive and you reprogrammed your mind and body to be able to do so and so it has been for every milestone you have achieved.

Many people get carried away by what is happening around them. Correct me, many people cannot manage their emotions in relation to what happens and, as we have said so far, it is not important what happens but how you react.

Experience is not what you face. We all face battles but we don't all get out of them equally. Here then we can say that experience is not what happens to a man but what a man does with what happens (cit. Aldouis Huxley). Are you complaining or looking for ways to exploit the situation? Do you stay focused on your goals or do you allow difficulties to prevail?

When you lose, don't miss the lesson.
(Dalai Lama)

If you don't understand that from everything that happens you can draw a lesson for your growth, how can you think of overcoming the same situation if it ever happens again in the future? The first goal we should set ourselves is to keep learning by lowering the mental barriers of our preconceptions.

We don't know everything, indeed, we know very little. We are 7 billion people on the planet and everyone would have to teach us something, each could offer us a different point of view from which to learn new information. This alone is enough for us to know that the emotions we are feeling, after all, are not the only ones that can be felt when faced with a given situation.

Our (emotional) intelligence lies in recognizing emotions, managing them, understanding which is best to indulge and which is better to subside. Knowing how to manage emotions allows us to better experience what, inevitably, we are required to experience. Emotions speak to us about us, thoughts, at times, just speak to us.

I try to explain myself better with this short story that Tiziano Terzani tells in one of his books:

A tiger had two followers: a leopard and a jackal. Whenever the tiger bit prey, she ate what she could and left the remains for the leopard and the jackal.

But one day it happened that the tiger killed three animals: one large, one medium and one small. "And now how do we divide them?" the tiger asked his two followers. "Simple, - replied the leopard, - you take the largest, I take the medium and the small one we give to the jackal".

The tiger said nothing, but with one paw it tore at the leopard. "So how do we divide them?" Asked the tiger again. "Oh, Majesty - answered the jackal, - you take the small piece for breakfast, you keep the big one for lunch and you eat the medium one for dinner".

The tiger was surprised. "Tell me, jackal, from whom did you learn so much wisdom?" The jackal hesitated for a while, then with the humblest air he managed to put on he replied: "From the leopard, Majesty."

The jackal, before answering, listened to his emotions, managed them, and intelligently governed the situation. His goal, in addition to eating, was to survive, so he responded according to the goals he had set.

Of all the experiences you have,
consider only the wisdom they contain.

(Mark Twain)

LEARNING TO MANAGE EMOTIONS: MEDITATION AND CONCENTRATION

There are countless mental strategies and techniques to learn to manage emotions but according to my experience (and not only) there is only one way to fulfill this task and that is meditation, the only useful way to train concentration.

Meditation is not only the ability to get away from one's thoughts by focusing on breathing (yes, I did it very quickly but try to follow me please), but it is also and above all the ability to think deeply and continuously about a single topic.

Do you know when a child is lost in his games and does not notice the passing of time and what is happening around him? Here, in that instant the child is meditating, his mind travels at very different frequencies than those of the mind of an adult who takes it out on the past and is anxious for the future.

Whenever you focus, place your attention on something, on a goal, and do it in a prolonged and concentrated way, here you are meditating, you are activating the power of intention. What happens is that you are channeling your energy (fragment of universal energy) towards a certain direction and the effect you will get will be the physical manifestation of the object / experience of your concentration.

You are the cause, life is the effect, but it is also true that the effect must first be experienced internally through the anticipated emotional experience of what will be. Where you focus your attention your intention is realized. What you think manifest.

This process of concentration activates the unconscious mind and allows you to observe emotions for what they are: bodies of energy that we can accept or reject. You, the sentient being who lives in the human body biological machine, can choose what to do with these energy bodies but you can only do it if you become aware of who you are. You are not the thoughts, you are not the emotion, you are not the body and you are not the mind. You are the Being, you are the light that creates, Soul.

Meditation and prayer are the fastest means we have to connect with the unconscious. Only when we are able to silence the mind can we capture the extrasensory intuitions, only in stillness can we access a different, higher awareness. The answers that the unconscious can offer you are very different from those offered by reason, but in order to access them you need to calm the mind, to re-tune it.

In this section, I don't want to suggest how to meditate , we have already done it previously, and I don't want to invite you to follow the guided relaxation to test the power of concentration first hand.

Rather I would like to invite you to write down your wishes and now I'll explain why.

But first of all let's stop calling them desires and let's call them for what they are, life goals, do you agree?

Identify and write down the goals you want to achieve on a piece of paper by dividing them as follows:

- one to three short-term goals (lead time from 1 to 12 months)
- one to three medium-term goals (1 to 3 years)
- one to three long-term goals (5 to 10 years).

Many personal growth gurus would invite you to write many more but I am from another school: if you put too much meat on the fire you will end up burning something, right?

After writing your goals, all you have to do is reread them several times a day focusing on them, dwelling on each one and expressing gratitude for the result achieved, then get excited as if everything had already happened. The secret is all in the as if! Try now what you will feel when it is. The unconscious does not recognize what is real from what is only imagined, it indiscriminately elaborates the images it receives in order for you to achieve them also on the physical plane.

The mental images wrapped in emotions create new furrows in the soil of your mind , new furrows where to sow the seeds of the reality that will manifest itself. The new mental images absorbed by the subconscious are able to generate new thoughts, therefore new actions, thus leading you to obtain new results.

As long as you walk the same roads you can't think of arriving in different places, right? Setting yourself goals and focusing on them with mind and heart allows you to turn at the right time to seize the most suitable opportunities to achieve the result.

Do you know when it is said that one is in the right place at the right time? Here, a piece is missing: one is in the right place at the right time only if he is the right person, and the right person is the one who has clearly in mind what he wants.

Luck is when the opportunity grasps your being prepared and you begin to be prepared the instant you have given a clear and precise shape to what it should be. It is no coincidence that we often say that what you already feel is what you get , right?

This exercise of transcribing goals and experiencing the sensations they will be able to bring in advance serves primarily to define a clear emotional destination within you . This will ensure that every time new emotions arise, your inner compass (by now trained) will know where to point. In order to manage emotions we must first understand the ones we prefer to feel, don't you think?

So if by chance you were wondering what being able to manage emotions with the transcription of your goals centered on you, I explained it to you : if you know where you want to go you can manage emotions better because you have an (emotional) direction to follow.

Usually, those who are unable to cope with events and let themselves be overwhelmed by their own emotions, are people who do not have a clear purpose, do not have clear goals in life, and I believe that first of all, before any other goal, it is appropriate for them to set out to achieve inner peace , this is a beautiful goal!

He who knows his goal feels strong; this strength makes him serene; this serenity ensures inner peace; only inner peace allows for deep reflection; deep reflection is the starting point of any success.

(Lao Tzu)

MEDITATION AND CONCENTRATION: THE TRUTH

Meditation and concentration are able to awaken the consciousness to the Truth in which we are inserted. And what is this Truth? The truth is that you project yourself outward, every moment you are in the continuous act of creating and recreating who you are and the world around you.

Meditation and concentration help you tune in to the reality you want to manifest and once this reality has come to life inside you, it can only manifest itself outside, it's inevitable!

Do not allow emotions to rule your existence, recognize them and manage them wisely. They are like the wind that blows but you are the sailor who maneuvers the sails to decide which direction to go! A life without goals is a life at the mercy of emotional winds. Goals are essentially used to help you move forward, to make you stronger and able to handle any event, which is why it is important that they are always present in your mind and heart ... a goal does not necessarily have to be achieved: often serves only as something to aim for.

Overcoming Obstacles To Achieve Discipline

I assure you that a life without obstacles is not a life! The human intellect is able to pose problems and find solutions, create alternatives, shape, generate art... all these things find an outlet in reality because reality presents challenges to overcome. If it hadn't been gravity you wouldn't have looked for a way to walk, so the birds wouldn't have found a way to use their wings. Difficulties sharpen our wits and push us to grow. Do you want to improve your life? Then it touches you! Find out how to overcome the obstacles that reality places on you. No obstacles, no evolution. Necessity drives us to do what we were born for, that is, to find solutions thanks to creativity, a capacity reserved for God ... and for us!

Every question expects an answer, every doubt requires clarification. The mind (when used correctly) is for this, to overcome the obstacles that present themselves to transform us into who we choose to be. The mind is creative . Each mental image assumed tends to manifest itself in its corresponding physical experience , whether you choose to visualize the future you want and identify with it, or whether you get emotionally involved in the gruesome images of a TG ... the (internal) emotion of today generates the (external) experience of tomorrow.

If you found yourself in a world of ready-to-eat meals, where all your needs were already solved, do you think you would set out to look for solutions? For what? Rather, you would run the risk of becoming lazy and turning off.

A goal that does not present difficulties to be pursued is not a goal, a prize without competition is not a prize, a victory without a battle is not a victory. Do you want to see the light? You have to go through the dark! Do you want to reach your goal? You have to face the obstacles that separate you from it, there is no alternative ...

Difficulty creates necessity, necessity forces you to innovate, to evolve towards a better version of yourself. Needs constitute demands and demands create action, which in turn leads to results.

The evolutionary process is constantly at work in building your future starting from the present you live. The thought / emotion asks through mental images, the action attracts, and you, Soul, receive the required experience.

It is no coincidence that we talk about the Law of Attraction , right?

If you had not encountered obstacles in your path you would not be as you are now. Every obstacle you passed yesterday allowed you to become who you are today.

To get started, you need to stop talking and take action.
(Walt Disney)

FACING OBSTACLES: THE MIND IS THE LIMIT

Whenever mother nature overcomes an obstacle it evolves. Do you remember the story of the squirrel who had to put his wings in order not to crash with every jump?

Every obstacle that Life encounters does not avoid it, it overcomes it. So do we humans ... when we don't give up! Those with greater resilience do better in this but also the less experienced, sooner or later, have to get used to the forced changes that this existence imposes, so they have to grow, evolve to a better version of themselves ... or succumb.

Jacques Lock, member of the Rockefeller Institute , through some experiments on plant parasites, showed how even the smallest beings adapt to the natural change that Life imposes and through which it thrives and spreads.

J.Lock placed vases with roses in front of windows. The aphids of the plant, as long as it was alive, drew nourishment from its sap. These aphids were wingless.

But the rose, left purposely without water, died after a few days. The aphids encountered an obstacle, that is, they had lost their nourishment. What happened was that these little beings grew temporary wings to fly away, towards the window light.

Mother Nature, your true Mother, knows no obstacles that cannot be overcome. If there are limits, the human mind creates them but they do not correspond to Truth. Limits are nothing but illusions that we believe to be real but the only reality is that limits do not exist, there are only objectives.

The obstacles that separate you from what you want to achieve are nothing more than the poles that show you the way to get to your destination. What you should ask yourself is whether you are willing to put in the effort to overcome them.

The instant you keep your focus on the goal, the solution appears by itself. The athlete sets the finish line. If he stared at the obstacle to climb over, he would trip over it ...

Obstacles are those scary things you see when you take your eyes off the goal.

(Henry Ford)

HOW NOT TO OVERCOME OBSTACLES: THE MIND MIND

Before discovering how to overcome obstacles, it seems appropriate to understand what not to do, what do you say? The way you use the mind determines the direction of your life but you are not the mind. The mind is a tool, you are the user. To control the mind you don't need the mind , you need presence.

When you are present in the now you have everything under control, when you get lost in the mental chatter you identify with the thought. But thought is an endless film projected onto the screen of your brain. You can observe it or you can get involved. You can check it or have it checked. You can silence the mind to find yourself or you can get lost in the inner dialogue until you never find yourself again, this is also a choice.

Imagine entering a huge, very crowded beer hall. Hear the background buzz of people talking, laughing, arguing, complaining, rejoicing ... every table is busy, everyone has their say, someone listens, the bartender yells at the colleague ... here, this is a snapshot of our mind when let it be. He chats constantly, one thought overlaps the other, a single voice multiplies itself infinitely, touching on numerous topics that nevertheless never ends.

Not being able to stop thinking is a terrible affliction, but we don't realize it because almost everyone suffers from it, so it's considered normal.
(Eckhart Tolle, The Power of Now)

Having said this, however, we can realize one thing, namely, that inside our head we are two. There are those who speak and there are those who listen. You are the one who listens and that if you only wanted to you could take over the reins of the dialogue, and then there is the other (the thinking entity) who, if left free, attacks with his usual blowjobs. Yes, usual blowjobs because his arguments are repeated like a broken record. In the incessant inner dialogue there is no creativity, no innovation, there is only a repetition of information already known, elaborated and reworked ad nauseam.

This incessant reprocessing of the data recorded in memory survives because an emotional memory is linked to each data. Whatever thought you have, any mental image of the past / future / present you can bring back, is intrinsically linked to an emotion otherwise it would not have been possible to engrave itself in your mind. We are emotional beings and it is not possible for us to live without feeling anything. If anything, emotions can be managed so as not to be overwhelmed by them but they cannot be canceled.

Inner dialogue is harmful, why? Because if it is not stopped, if we do not stop identifying with it, we will be overwhelmed by losing the opportunity to hear our true voice, the voice of the Soul. Soul expresses itself through the sixth sense, intuition, by means of sensations, visions, ideas, flashes of genius ... capturing these energy bodies is possible in the instant we remain present in the now. And presence means silence ...

If you can grasp the present moment, if you can change it by changing your perception, you will have obtained the key to consciously change your life. Change who you are right now and you will have changed everything. Come back to the here & now and overcoming obstacles will be like breathing, a natural process.

So here is a short list of things that the background chatter of your mind leads you to do that do not allow you to overcome obstacles:

- continue to remain in a state of fear
- keep the guilt alive
- attacking and defending stereotyped, harmful and little thought habits
- refuse to have self-discipline capable of creating / manifesting the new
- avoid emotions such as love, joy, gratitude and sharing
- fuel complaints and pessimism
- blaming and judging the work of others and one's own
- feel a sense of inferiority
- find excuses to justify yourself and not take full responsibility for yourself

This list could get even longer, right? I want to close this paragraph with a short video. This is a scene from the movie "The Neverending

Story". The unfortunate Artax allowed sadness to take over... here's another thing we can't allow to happen to us if we want to overcome our obstacles!

HOW TO OVERCOME OBSTACLES: EVOLUTION AND NECESSITY

As said before, our task is to reduce the obstacles of life to understand that they are nothing but necessities useful for our progress. And it is not what kind of adversity we face is important, but how we face it. It's not what happens that makes the difference but how you react to what happens.

Had Artax been more motivated he would not have collapsed. Yes, I know, we are talking about a horse, but try to understand... if we lose sight of our goals we lose sight of ourselves. It doesn't matter what happens outside. Reality does not exist, there is only perception and the perception of what happens is under your direct control. How do you want to get involved in an event? What do you choose to place your mental energy on?

If you allow the outside world to manipulate your attention, your emotionality, therefore your mental images, you are literally leaving the reprogramming of your unconscious paradigm in the hands of others and the results could be catastrophic.

Are you going through a difficult time? You are scared? Do you feel helpless? Do the obstacles seem out of your reach? Good! This is where you need to pay more attention. Deliberately choose the information you want to feed on because every seed you plant in your unconscious will bear fruit. Now more than ever you need to focus on what you want, not what you don't want.

There is only one thing that you need to remember before discovering how to overcome obstacles and it is this: every information (mental / emotional image) that you insert into your brain is metabolized by the subconscious mind which, sooner or later, will offer you a result of the same nature in the form of physical experience.

I know that advice is not offered if it is not requested but for once listen to me: do you want to watch television? Watch it as long as you want as long as you leave it off! That damn appliance is capable of brainwashing you by losing sight of your mission. And do you know what your mission is? Love, create and share in love, to be useful to you and to others. The purpose of existence is to evolve and the purpose of this evolution is you .

So, how to overcome the obstacles:

Choose information that is useful for your well-being and purpose. The unconscious mind is constantly receiving, it constantly absorbs all kinds of signals that the conscious mind sends it. You have the duty and the right to choose what to feed it with knowing full well that you will reap the benefits of what you are sowing.

Stay focused on the goal.

Don't lose sight of your mission: to love, create, share . If you stay focused on who you are, everything will be fine. Don't get distracted and don't let the outside world interrupt your path. The steps you take in the most difficult moments are also the most impactful ones. He who sows in tears will reap in joy (psalm 126)

Be grateful for the difficulties.

Each obstacle carries with it the seed of tomorrow's fortune. Beyond all difficulties there is a dream that asks for nothing more than to be lived. So thank the opportunity you have to face the challenges of living and that allow you to continually evolve towards who you are wanting to be, towards a better version of you.

Be compassionate to those who can't.

Many people next to you could interfere with your purpose, you know that. Be deaf to complaints and blame, just offer the world the best you can. There is a saying that says what you do speaks so loudly that I can't hear what you say . Here! The only way you can lend a hand to those who cannot keep the right course is to make your contribution with deeds, not words. Don't get lost in useless ticks that solve nothing, take action!

OBSTACLES: YOUR RENAISSANCE

The art of living consists in making the most of good out of the most evil.

(Joaquim Maria Machado de Assis)

There was a historical period in which we experienced demographic, economic and cultural deterioration… no, I'm not talking about today. I refer to the dark ages, to the Middle Ages. The Roman Empire collapsed and Europe plunged into a nightmare.

But do you know what happened at the end of this dark period? It happened that many relied on the light they had inside and this is how the Renaissance began.

This historical period radically changed the paradigms of the human being and saw the flourishing of artistic and cultural disciplines, especially in Italy, the cradle of this evolution of consciousness. This rebirth led the human being to conceive the world and himself in a different way but I'm sure you know all this. The Renaissance began because darkness had allowed light to spread.

Obstacles serve to improve your life, not the other way around. Even if everything seems to be going wrong, remember that spring always follows winter. If you like rainbows you have to accept the rain, if you want to see the stars embrace the night, if you want to admire the rising of a new dawn cross the darkness keeping in mind your purpose.

Every tree that grows and blooms is nothing more than the explosion of a previously planted seed. What fruits do you want to harvest tomorrow? What seeds are you planting today? Whatever is happening out there you have no reason to stop creating, loving and sharing.

Spiritual Therapy & Mental Discipline

All diseases are psychosomatic and are the result of incorrect mental / emotional behavior as well as a harmful lifestyle. The section could end here because in this sentence there is everything you need to know to not get sick. But let's go deeper: today we talk about illness and the unconscious.

The mind is the creator and the only creator. Who you are today, the results you get, and your weight, your finances... everything is a reflection of how you have used your mind up to now. You are who you create. When you correct your mind, everything else is corrected.

I'm not a doctor, I want to clarify it, and do you know why? Because the topic we are going to deal with today will find many disagree, I already know. And I'll tell you more! It will be more than normal that many will resent what I write. The reason? In the West, we have been conditioned to think of disease in a certain way. If you made the things you read in this section public in another socio-cultural context, they would surely find much more approval. Patience! I write what I think and what I write I share. I correct myself: I write what I understand...

I don't think there is a pill for every disease, as common thinking would have us believe. I rather believe in the law of causality, the law of cause and effect, where the effects we suffer are the result of the causes we have put into play. Illness does not happen, it does happen, as does health. Everything is the result of something and if we don't like the result we have to change the cause that triggered it.

It does not seem appropriate to me to start from the origins to deal with this topic. I mean, I'm not going to explain to you that if you smoke, eat out of proportion and don't move, you can never be healthy, right?

Life is on your side the instant you are on its side. Take care of the biological organism that has been entrusted to you that is the mind / body system you are using to enjoy this journey, and you will see that you will not know disease.

When you eat in fast food restaurants are you loving yourself? Are you taking care of yourself? When you are filled with anger, hatred, envy, are you loving yourself? When you go looking for injustices to complain about your situation are you taking care of your well-being? Loving oneself means calibrating one's behavior, resizing one's habits, in such a way as to get the best out of oneself, in such a way as not to cause any harm to one's person, both internally and externally.

So today I'm not going to tell you what to do or not to do to be in excellent health. I'll assume that you already know what to avoid in order not to harm yourself.

What I want to talk to you about today is how and why your unconscious mind organizes the health of your body. As mentioned above, whatever results you get are the fruit of the seeds you planted inside of you.

BEHAVIORAL MEDICINE

With this section I want to address first of all to those who already know the rules of good behavior in the name of psycho-physical well-being but who despite everything find themselves suffering from different types of malaise.

It is often not enough to exercise and eat properly to stay healthy. We know it. Often what makes us sick are anger, sorrow, fear ... low vibrations!

In fact, the body does not get sick, it simply reflects the condition of our predominant mood. And the predominant mood is the result of the unconscious paradigm we are using to interface with the world out there. Yes, because if you haven't figured it out yet, it's a chaos out there, an apparent chaos in perfect order, and nothing makes sense except what you give it.

Just as when we feel ashamed we turn red, so every emotion affects our body. Anger bites the stomach, love opens the heart wide, jealousy compresses it, fear takes away energy from the kidneys ... and these emotions can not only be experienced in the present moment, but they can become unconscious predominant emotions the instant you dedicate them most attention (perhaps by repeatedly remembering the experience that generated them) or if you experience them in a traumatic way through some event that has shocked you. Do you remember how the unconscious works?

If you continuously feel gratitude during the day, gratitude would become your predominant state of being. The unconscious mind would recognize this emotion as the most suitable to face life and consequently it would predispose the entire body to this frequency, a frequency of love, health and well-being.

Just as cancer cannot develop in an alkaline environment, disease cannot manifest itself in an inhospitable body. And the body is inhospitable to malaise when traveling at high frequencies / vibrations.

All diseases are tuned to the low frequencies, the same ones that are generated by fear, anger, sadness. High frequencies (love, gratitude, joy, enthusiasm, etc ...) do not allow your body to get sick. How come when you are grateful you can't be sad?!? Two vibrations of different types cannot coexist. Have you ever seen a person who is enthusiastic and depressed at the same time?

There was a time when I did not deal with certain issues but from the moment I had the possibility of choice I no longer wanted to entrust myself exclusively to traditional medicine. As a child, of course, I too was indoctrinated to the dogmas of our culture. I haven't had a cold for many years now and not because I was lucky, but because I corrected what was wrong with nutrition, behavior and thinking. The last fever I remember lasted an hour. To get it through I ran 10 km.

I'm not telling you that this is the solution to all evils, mind you. If you're out of practice, running will only hurt you. What I want to emphasize is that there is a different way to feel good than what is proposed to us, I call it behavioral prevention and we start by making this belief our own: the disease is not a possibility, it is a result whose cause originated in the my mind. The state of health of the body is directly proportional to the love that I express towards me through thoughts, emotions, actions.

Now I repeat what you have often already read on these pages but if I repeat it it is only because it is absolutely important to remember it:

we are vibrational beings embedded in a vibrational reality. Everything affects each other. We attract to us all that is on the same vibrational frequency. The physical body welcomes everything that resonates with its energy. When you are afraid of getting sick, you just tune in to the disease itself and predispose the body to welcome / activate the parasite / malaise. Fear weakens, love heals.

The medicine industry doesn't care that you are okay, it doesn't care that you are aware of how it works, it cares about your fear, without it it wouldn't bill. You are useful to him if you get sick, not if you stay healthy. The media convey low frequencies influencing the masses and the masses get sick. But we will not talk about this in this section. We have to keep the frequencies high, right?

DISEASE AND UNCONSCIOUS: THE WILL TO LIVE

Let's get back to us. Unconscious and disease, what connection exists between the two?

Health is the main factor of happiness. If you were not in good health you could not enjoy anything, not your loved ones, not your money, not your freedom, nothing at all. A happy mind lives in a healthy body , a sick body hosts an unhappy mind. Sadness weakens you, happiness strengthens your immune system.

But do you know what is the factor that affects the most in the recovery of a sick person? It is the will to live! People with the same disease do not necessarily have the same chance of recovery. There are people who want to heal and continue living, there are others who break down and lose all desire for life. The consequences of the two mental attitudes are obviously different.

I'll tell you a true story ...

It is the story of a man in his fifties who loses his job. He has no family, he lives alone and the only way to feel useful to society is to occupy that office as an employee. He dedicates his life to work, makes him happy, makes him feel fulfilled. In work it finds its purpose.

One day the company he works for closes. He is redeemed. In six months of redundancy, he finds no one willing to hire him. He goes into depression, he never leaves the house anymore.

It's January and a chill forces him to bed with the flu. The flu lasts for 3 weeks. It does not pass. His condition worsens. Doctors don't understand, he probably does. After a month of flu the man dies.

Cause of death? Officially it is a weakening of the lymphatic system. But that was only a consequence. The reality is that the man, a friend of my family, had lost the will to live. Man had nothing more to cling to, nothing more to love, nothing more to continue living for. He hadn't understood that if he wanted to start over, he had to start over from himself. He had to start loving himself.

The mental attitude of a sick person determines his recovery (placebo effect, nocebo effect), any doctor can confirm this but I guess you already know it.

Everyone's life force resides not in the body but in the mind. Puny people managed to survive the concentration camps, others more robust did not. And the will to live is not something that we study, it is something that resides in the deepest part of us, resides in the unconscious, is called the survival instinct and is as strong as our love for Life is strong.

The unconscious has absolute control over the functions and conditions of the body, so there is no situation that the unconscious cannot control if this is our will and the will to live is nothing but the love we feel towards us themselves.

Self-love corrects harmful mental / emotional behaviors as well as actions. Only by learning to love ourselves will we be able to love others and it will be the love towards others that will spread and then return to the origin, giving us more and more Life.

The unconscious, as extensively described in YOU ARE WHO CREATE , can always be controlled by the power of suggestion. Which means that the desire to heal is all that the unconscious needs in order to help the organic system free itself from evil.

When the mind is healthy, the body is healthy. And when the body is functioning regularly then it resists the germs of the disease as well as its negativity by not being in resonance with its vibration. But if the resistance is weakened by negative emotional reactions, then both the health of the body and the mind are very easily lost.

Emotional disturbances disrupt the balanced functioning of the human organism and emotional disturbances are not necessarily only those that occur following events of the present moment. Indeed, to influence our state of health the most are those disorders that are buried in our memory, in the unconscious, concerning past experiences.

Here is a short exercise to clear your unconscious mind of old emotional residues.

Is there any unpleasant event in your past that can only arouse in you those negative emotions you felt then? If so, then you are faced with an emotional residue, an emotional scar that has never healed.

Try to relive that event but try to observe it in the third person. Observe yourself then as you relive the situation. Observe without judging or identifying yourself, as if it were a silent black and white film projected on a screen. Look at the past. There is nothing of that event anymore except in your mind. If it has happened it means that there is a lesson to be learned but to do so you have to put your emotional system out of the way. Analyze it coldly.

What happened? What have you learned? Don't look for the culprits or those responsible, it doesn't help you. Instead, try to relive the situation by replacing the old feelings with a new understanding, the understanding of forgiveness, then forgive the protagonists of that event, including yourself. That event is a moment of life and as such it needs your blessing. Protect it, keep it, love it. If it happened, you see that it needed to happen to teach you something. True failure is not the negative event itself, failure is if we learn nothing from it, we do not learn to love ourselves more. Failure is if a better human being does not come out of that event.

When you have faith in the success of something you don't care about the hesitation that fear offers you, or am I wrong? Act with courage, with love, with faith, defending your vision because you feel that not only is it possible, but it is inevitable.

It has been proven that faith is one of the factors that most affects the healing of the body (and the success of our projects). Don't get me wrong, I'm not telling you to have faith in God, mother nature or Life. We are not talking about this now.

I am simply suggesting that you have faith in healing. Healing is the natural process by which nature is self-fulfilling and self-correcting. Healing doesn't happen the instant we insert doubt / fear energy into our experience.

Trusting to heal means having a clear and clear mental image of oneself in the conditions we expect to occur. The mental image you have of yourself is reflected in reality.

If you were afraid you would not be able to create an image of yourself in perfect physical shape. Rather you would project a future filled with the bad things that could happen. Conversely, if you felt love, you would be able to anticipate the feeling of joy and gratitude for the impending healing.

Jesus thanked the Father for the miracles that occurred even before they occurred, do you understand what I have told you? The anticipated emotion is the essence of your desire. The unconscious mind believes in the visions you offer it and on which you linger with sufficient emotional charge (no matter if negative or positive) and will do everything to realize them on the physical plane.

This is what spiritual therapy is all about. Therapy that if accompanied by a healthy lifestyle and proper nutrition can only guarantee you a good health of mind and body. We always reap what we sow and our unconscious is very fertile ground as you well know.

ILLNESS DOES NOT EXIST: LOVED YOU NOT TO SICK

Do you remember what the fourth Hermetic Law says? The Law of Polarity ? It briefly says this: everything moves on a scale, from the lowest value to the highest value.

If you asked a physicist to describe cold to you, he would answer you like this: cold does not exist as it is not measurable. What we can measure is the heat. When it is cold, there is simply a lower level of heat. Heat is energy, cold is nothing.

And the same thing goes for the disease. It is nothing more than a lack of health. Poverty is a lack of wealth, fear is a lack of love, darkness is a lack of light, etc ...

It's like there are knobs for everything to adjust the intensity, have you ever thought about that? And the main volume to be adjusted, the one that consequently amplifies everything else, is the volume of Love towards oneself. When the love knob is at its maximum, everything else tends to increase accordingly, right?

Life does not want disease for you, it wants life, it wants to experience itself through itself, through you. He doesn't want to turn you off, he wants to enlighten you so that you can spread a little light around you too and to do that he needs you to choose to love yourself. How do you know if you are loving yourself? Simple: are your choices in favor of your well-being?

I conclude by bringing back the Truth that you would do well to embrace. Read the sentences that follow, aloud, perhaps looking yourself in the eyes in the mirror, until you feel that you firmly believe in what you are saying. Just as it is true that water is wet, so these words will resonate with who you really are by vibrating your innermost part. Because deep down, let's face it, YOU know who you are: you are who you create .

Stress Management for Mental Discipline

Do you know what stresses us the most? It is not what we do to respond to the tasks of life that stress us, rather it is what we expect to happen if we do not act to stress ourselves. Was I unclear? Let's try again: going to work tomorrow morning, facing the day, doing the tasks that are due to us and then going home are not stressful facts. What stresses us most is the thought we have now of having to do those things tomorrow and do them again the day after tomorrow. In the last section, we saw how worry is only an automatic response to an external or mental stimulus, today we see how stress management starts from understanding that it is we who anticipate the tension of something that does not yet happen.

Do you know what caused your stress? It was an evaluation thought that you previously generated about something. Stress arises when something is bothering you. If something is bothering you, it means that you are giving it mental and emotional attention. This attention, when you go on for a long time, becomes stress. This, in short, is what happens.

If you don't think about it and just act, you don't get stressed, do you? Apparently it is the thought that stresses us. What we do during the day, if anything, can tire us, not generate stress, they are two completely different things. It is no coincidence that the most stressed people are those who hold sedentary roles. Their body is unable to discharge the mental and emotional energy of the attention they have devoted to a particular matter and so they build up tension.

And have you ever noticed that the word attention contains within it the word tension? It is disguised, instead of an S it has a Z. Stress does the same: it disguises itself as normality ...

Tension is who you think you should be. Peace is who you are.
(Chinese proverb)

And as you know, first I make you aware of the problem, I offer you the tools to recognize it, then I suggest how to deal with it. We cannot defeat what we do not know, much less we can eliminate something we do not know exists.

There are people who do not even notice that they are stressed but if you point out their state of health and the answers they offer to the outside they take a step back and wonder how they did not notice that they got to that point. But that's another story ...

Stress can affect everyone... everyone except children! And do you know why? Children are carefree, carefree. Their minds are limited to offering serene responses to events occurring in the present moment and are not used to facing concerns about the future.

And what did Jesus say about it? If you want to live in the kingdom of God, you must return as a child! The kingdom of God is nowhere to be found, it is not in heaven and you do not reach it after death. The kingdom of God is this moment, the here and now, the only place in space and time where miracles, or changes of state, can occur .

When in your life you have managed to do something incredible, when you have experienced a moment of intense enthusiasm, when you were in the height of your joy and energy, where were you with your mind if not in the present moment? The Guided Meditation is a valuable aid for ricentrarci, but often not enough. There are occasions where our presence is necessary and we cannot afford to be absent. So how does stress management happen? Let's start to understand it with this short story that newsletter subscribers already know ...

HOW MUCH DOES YOUR GLASS OF WATER WEIGH?

It is said that a professor of Psychology from the University of Berkely entered the classroom with a glass of water in his hand.

In the classroom, rumors began. Some thought that the teacher wanted to talk about optimism, about a glass half full and half empty. But what he simply asked was:

"How much does this glass of water weigh"?

The students tried to answer: someone said 200 grams, someone else 300, 350, 400 ...

"The absolute weight of the glass of water is irrelevant", replied the professor, "what matters most is how long you hold it up.

Lift it up for a minute, and you won't have any problems!
Lift it for an hour, and you'll end up with a sore arm.
Lift it up for a whole day, and you will end up with a paralyzed arm!

In each of these three cases the weight of the glass did not change! Yet, the more time passes, the heavier the glass seems to become... Stress and worries are like this glass of water.

Small or large, what matters is how much time we dedicate to them. If we dedicate the minimum time necessary to them, our mind is not affected.

If we start thinking about it several times during the day, our mind starts to get tired and nervous. If we constantly think about our worries, our mind is paralyzed!

To find peace of mind, you must learn to let go of stress and worries. You must learn to devote as little time to them as possible, focusing your attention on what you want, not what you don't want!

You have to learn how to put the glass of water down! "

Rest every now and then; a field that has rested yields an abundant harvest. (Ovid)

LIFE IS REALIZED WITHOUT STRESS

Do you know what our drama is? It is that we feel obliged to live, or rather, to survive. In reality, no one is forcing us to stay here. If we wanted to, we could end it at any moment, have you ever thought about it? But what is that force that pushes us to move forward, that pushes us to continue through difficulties, making us always winners? Because in the end this is who you are: a winner, a survivor of the life that happens. You have always won and you will do it until the end of your days. Events can bend you but not break you. Either way, you will

94

stay on your feet, whether you decide to complain, play the victim, or roll up your sleeves and take full responsibility for your life.

But the truth is, we don't have to live. We choose to live, every day. Those who choose to end it do the same and, on the contrary, choose to stop living. The thought of death cannot frighten him because in it he idealizes the salvation of himself, the end of suffering. When we die, worries cease to exist. Suicides take this path convinced that it is the definitive solution to problems that are in reality temporary but that they perceive as insurmountable, they see no alternatives.

The spirit of survival fails, or maybe it gets stronger, it depends on how we choose to see the issue, or not? Does the spirit want to free itself from the shackles of earthly dramas and therefore choose to elevate itself by freeing itself from the flesh? This happens when living becomes an unsustainable, unbearable effort. But living doesn't have to be an effort, don't you think? Why should there be tension in living? Why do we generate stress? Because, in fact, we pay constant attention to obstacles and we stop seeing the beyond , where the obstacle has already been overcome.

You are the only problem you will ever have. You are the only solution. (Bob Proctor)

Let's try to observe nature. For an animal, for a plant, continuing to live is something spontaneous, it is not a stretch. In Chinese, the word nature is ziran. But this term means much more. Ziran is a key concept of Taoism and literally means "naturally; spontaneously; freely; obviously; no doubt; what happens by itself '".

When we force ourselves to live, when we force ourselves to face events with discontent rather than accept them, when we choose to perceive the weight of Life rather than its flowering, we do nothing but oppose what happens by itself . We interrupt the spontaneous development of what already is and create inner malaise.

In the instant that we allow Life to happen without judging it instead, everything is back in order and everything is realized in ways that we would never have thought of. The caterpillar becomes a butterfly, the sprout pierces the earth, the unborn child sees the light... all these things happen from uncomfortable positions but they happen! And these things happen not because they have to be done, but because they are ...

The student had just been beaten in a fight with a fellow student. Disappointed by the umpteenth defeat, he tried to understand the reasons,
so he turned to his Master:

- "Master, once again I have been defeated, something is missing in my technique."
- "What causes the defeat is not the lack of technique, but the reason why you want to win and therefore clash.
- When you are at peace with yourself, when you don't have to get something that you get anxious about, you can never be defeated.
- Go and keep training. "

The boy turned and went back to his partner
to continue the challenge with himself.

STRESS MANAGEMENT: 4 STRATEGIES

Forgive the long preamble but you know very well that the clearer we do, the better we see the view. It is one thing to be inside a labyrinth and look for a way out, another thing is to be able to see the labyrinth from above to find the best path to solve it, right? Here are 4 strategies that will help you manage stress:

Delay response to events.

If you find that life's chores are draining your energy, stop for a moment. Write down all the tasks you have to do, in this way the attention you dedicate to them is limited and your mind can stop thinking about it, so much by now you have taken note, nothing escapes you anymore. Once you've written down your assignments, take your time and accurately choose the right time to tackle them. It is not about procrastinating but calmly deciding the best time to intervene. Delaying the response, choosing when this should happen, allows you to detach yourself from the tension that the thought of it carries with it. And do you know why? Because you are deliberately choosing not to obey the automatic mental and emotional response you usually have, the one that generates worry, anxiety and stress. You are literally taking back control of yourself. You choose when and how to act, events do not choose for you.

Relieve muscle tension.

Response means tension. Lack of response means relaxation. Turbulent feelings such as fear, anxiety, anger, hostility, insecurity, are caused by the responses you offer, not what happens. When the muscles are completely relaxed it is impossible to experience these feelings. These feelings are nothing more than the result of preparing for action . When muscles prepare for action, they generate tension, which in turn results in emotion. The relaxation of the muscles produces a mental abandonment, a mental abandonment generates a relaxed attitude. Relaxation is a natural tranquilizer that protects us from stress.

Create a mental refuge.

It doesn't matter where you go or where you are. If you do not find peace within you, no place can give it to you. People seek refuge by escaping from their everyday life. Houses in the countryside, beaches, mountains… these are all places that should relax us but if we keep certain thoughts alive inside, going to these places will not bring any benefit. Marcus Aurelius used to say that nowhere, however quiet and far from annoyance it may be, can a man find refuge as in his own soul, especially when he has thoughts in his depths such that only by examining them can he immediately find tranquility: and I affirm that tranquility is nothing but a good ordering of the mind. Constantly, therefore, allow yourself this sort of retreat and renew yourselves.

With your imagination, you can create a mental refuge to go to for peace of mind. Just as you have furnished your living room, decorate this imaginary room. Put in it anything that can bring you well-being, a bookcase, a comfortable armchair, a window overlooking the sea ... this place is nowhere but in you. Use it whenever you feel the need, it is an excellent remedy to detach yourself from the accumulated tensions. Imagine entering it, smelling it, feeling its silence. The more details you use in this view, the more benefit you will derive. The more times a day you allow yourself to take advantage of this place, the less stress you will accumulate. And who said that to go on vacation you have to wait for the summer? This place is always at your disposal and it only takes a few moments to enter.

Reset the stress counter.

If you take a trip by car and you want to know the distance you will travel, bring the odometer to zero, right? Do the same with you! Reset your counter! Every time you allow yourself to enter your mental refuge, just this happens: you reset the odometer of the tension. When you go from one task to another, from one situation to another, from one state to another, you need different resources. Your mental structure and attitude change with changing events. You adapt to what happens, you model yourself on the different experiences you face, and based on what happens you use resources or not, you need or not a certain type of mental and emotional reactions. This is why it is important to reset your approach to life whenever life around you changes. Think if every time you come home from work you bring with you all the thoughts and moods that your working day has offered you!?! You would argue with your partner, you would not stand your children, you would argue with the neighbor who makes more noise than usual... and this is because your internal counter has not been reset and continues to accumulate tension. You are mentally and emotionally reliving situations that are no longer present and you are reviving yourself in the present with the same type of energy used previously, a counterproductive energy and no longer suitable for the moment ... a little out of place, isn't it?

Before closing I would like to summarize what we have said about stress management with this short tip: choose to be fully involved in the present moment, whatever you are doing, whether you are choosing to relax and not give space to burdens and duties, whether you are choosing to act / react to events. Be present with your mind and heart, but above all, be appropriate to the circumstances. And instead of calling it duty or work, realize that you are just playing a beautiful game, a game called Life! To win you have to be present, to win you have to live the only time possible: the now.

Inferiority Complex & Mental Discipline

95% of people are convinced that they are not worth enough to deserve more. The fact is that we are all hypnotized by the truths we tell ourselves about ourselves. What you convince yourself of becomes real and most of the time these beliefs are difficult to recognize, they are unconscious, you don't even know you have them but they direct your life. Do you want to understand which beliefs reside in your unconscious? Look at your results, they are a perfect expression of your internal paradigm, a reflection of who you are if you prefer. Look at your relationships, your weight , your finances ... everything is an expression of the belief / paradigm you have embraced.

The inferiority complex is the product of one or more disempowering beliefs that we have accepted or created on our behalf and certainly cannot lead those who suffer from it to achieve their goals. If you think you are not worth enough why should you think you deserve plenty ? How could you find the grit needed to push yourself and achieve the results you aspire to?

So: how to cure the inferiority complex? We will see it shortly. Meanwhile, I will reveal a little secret that few know and those few who know it certainly do not come to tell you: any belief you want to embrace is pure illusion, an illusion that will become reality over time. This means that even the inferiority complex is only an illusion and is not based on anything tangible. It is just a thought and as such it can be replaced with another. And guess what, you choose your thoughts! But let's take it one step at a time ...

THE POWER OF ILLUSION

An illusion is nothing but a perception distorted by an error of the senses or of the mind. Or at least, this is the description that we find written in the dictionaries.

But the mind works through images and for it any image becomes real the instant we offer it our psychic and emotional energy. The mind does not distinguish what is real from what is not and it is precisely for this reason that we can say that the reality we are experiencing is pure illusion, a projection of our mind.

The verb 'deluding' has been given a purely negative meaning. Deluding yourself about something usually also reveals the other side of the coin, which is disappointment, or am I wrong? We are under the illusion that we can achieve something only to discover that it was not true. That girl deceived my hopes, the professor deceived me into thinking he was promoting myself, the dealer deceived me that the car was in good condition... and so on.

The positive effect of the illusion is rarely taken into consideration. And to think that illusionists and hypnotists use the power of illusion to entertain people or to heal them from the useless truths they have been told. I repeat: any illusion becomes real to the mind (otherwise it would not have been called an illusion). And why not delude yourself of something useful that can make us progress rather than suffer? Mental training is for this.

Did I mention that hypnotists and illusionists harness the power of illusion? Here then is a real fact that will make you understand in all respects what the mind is able to do when it deludes itself about something that is not there ... but that it exists for it!

In 1942, during the Second World War, General Rommel (better known as "the fox of the desert") was in charge of the Nazi troops in Africa. He was feared for his infallible strategic skills and rumor had paranormal powers that could predict the enemy's moves.

Nothing is easier than deluding oneself because
man believes what he desires is true.

(Demosthenes)

The illusion is not something true or not true, it is simply a thought that can replace another. If you think you can't achieve the result you want, you are deluding yourself that you can't. Your new illusion could instead be this: the result I want to achieve is the inevitable consequence of my action and it cannot help but reveal itself because if I insist and resist, I reach and conquer! Do you remember what Henry Ford said: whether you think you can or you can't, you will still be right! So all heard and done!

COMPLEX OF INFERIORITY AND HYPNOSIS

Those suffering from the inferiority complex have been hypnotized by a wrong opinion about themselves. And it doesn't matter if this false idea of self has been passed on to him by the media, parents or teachers. What is important to understand is that this idea steers the compass of his life.

He firmly believes in the veracity of this idea and as long as he remains firm in his conviction, this idea can only be reflected on the outside. Like attracts like.

Muhammad Ali, one of the greatest boxers ever, understood the power of self-hypnosis well and certainly didn't win matches because he felt inferior to his opponents. Do you know what he thought of himself? Here are some of his best-known quotes:

It's just my job. The grass grows, the birds fly, the waves wet the sand. And I win matches.

If you just dream of beating me, you better wake up and apologize.

I am the greatest, I said it before I even knew I was.

I am the greatest. Not only do I KO them, but I also choose the round.

Muhammad Ali was convinced (hypnotized) that he was the best... and he has become! The repetition of affirmations leads to belief and when the belief becomes a deep belief things start to happen.

When a person is hypnotized (whether he hypnotizes himself, knowingly or not, or someone else does) he is able to do surprising things because he is convinced of the truthfulness of the statements his mind receives and when this happens the person is behaves differently, thinks differently, and therefore gets different results. The power of hypnosis is nothing more than the power of believing and we all believe in something, that's why we can say that we are all hypnotized by the idea of the self that we have created.

The good news is that this idea we have about ourselves can be replaced at any time with a new one in case we don't like it ...

For what it's worth, it's never too late, or in my case too early, to be who you want to be. There is no time limit, start when you want, you can change or stay as you are, there is no rule in that. We can experience everything for the best or for the worst, I hope you experience everything to the fullest, I hope you can see amazing things, I hope you can always have new emotions, I hope you can meet people with different points of view, I hope you can be proud of your life and if you find that you are not, I hope you find the strength to start from scratch.

During sessions or hypnosis shows you can witness real miracles. Some examples: stuttering and shy people are convinced that they have no difficulty in dialogue and here we can hear them speak fluently in front of an audience, normally gifted people are convinced that they have more strength than usual and here they are lifting weights out of the ordinary for any individual. Hypnosis did not add anything to these people, rather it eliminated that limitation that lay in the idea of self they were relying on.

But hypnosis also works in reverse, for example when athletes with strong physique are convinced that they have no skills to lift a pencil. Here then you can see them in serious difficulty in the vain attempt to lift a weight of a few grams. In this case the hypnosis did not weaken the athlete, it simply pushed him to work against himself.

The idea of the ego is distorted and he believes that he is no longer able to lift any weight. The idea of "you can't do it" takes over on an unconscious level, regardless of the person's conscious will, and leads him to defeat himself by preventing him from expressing and putting his full potential into play.

However, nothing magical happens during hypnosis. Simply the hypnotist convinces the victim that now they can or cannot do something and urges them to move forward on that idea. Energy, the ability to do or not to do something, was already inherent in people but they were unable to reach it or oust it because they were unaware.

Long story short: within you exists the capacity and energy to express your full potential and to unearth the wonders you desire. Within you there is the possibility to do things you never thought you could do and this possibility becomes real the instant you change the limiting opinions to which you have made yourself hypnotizable, opinions like I can't, I'm not worthy, I'm not capable , I do not deserve it ... These are just opinions and since opinions become reality for your mind the only way you can change what you don't like about yourself is to hypnotize yourself to something more useful.

INFERIORITY COMPLEX: HOW TO TREAT IT

Each of us is inferior in something to someone else but if you judge a fish by its ability to climb trees it will spend its whole life believing that it is stupid (Einstein quote).

For example, I can't lift two hundred kilos like Arnold Schwarzenegger, I can't speak and act in French like Alain Delon, I'm unable to tango like Miguel Zotto, I'm unable to sculpt like Michelangelo or paint like Caravaggio. This makes me inferior to them only in specific abilities but it does not make me inferior to them as a person. On the other hand, there will be things that I can do excellently and they don't.

It is not being aware of a particular deficit compared to someone else that creates the inferiority complex but it is the feeling of inferiority that is generated that manages to interfere with our life.

And when does the feeling of inferiority arise? It arises when we judge and measure ourselves not on our model but on the model that someone else (religion, media, parents, teachers ...) has offered us. When this happens we always have the worst and do you know why? Because we begin to think that we are not enough to deserve the best, to deserve success and happiness.

I didn't come into the world to compete with anyone. Anyone who wants to compete with me loses his time. I'm in the world to compete with myself. Overcoming my limits, overcoming my fears, fighting against my defects, overcoming my difficulties and running in search of my goals. And all this already takes me a lot of time!

(A. De Mello)

When this happens it means that we have let ourselves be hypnotized by the mistaken idea that we must be a certain way or that we must be like everyone else. But how can we be like everyone else if we are all different? You already understand for yourself that building your life based on this idea is crazy.

Will those suffering from the inferiority complex try to reach the supposed level of the model they have considered and what happens?

It happens that to reach that level it needs to be superior and the most common risk is that the inferiority complex turns into a superiority complex. But superiority and inferiority are two sides of the same coin... yes, a counterfeit medal!

You cannot be inferior to someone else. Much less can you be superior. You can simply be YOU, this is the truth, and I assure you that you are perfect just the way you are. Individuality is what makes us special. Trying to conform to a model makes us lose our uniqueness.

And do you know how to get rid of the false idea of inferiority? We need to release the tension it has generated, we need to relax.

The opinions and beliefs you have embraced in your life have become yours without any kind of effort. You have been hypnotized while you were in complete relaxation, from when you were in the cradle until now, and that is why it is essential to return to the same condition to be despotized.

An expert connoisseur of autosuggestion , discovered that the efforts to obtain something are the main cause for which it cannot be obtained. On the contrary, if we prepare ourselves in a relaxed way to reach that something (as if it already belongs to us), our action will no longer be a continuous effort but a simple flow that will inevitably lead us to the goal.

Suggestions (ideal goals) must arise spontaneously if they want to be efficient.

(Emile Coué)

According to Coué, the manifestation of our inner energy is subordinated to the law of reversed effort which states that when will and imagination are in conflict, the imagination invariably wins the battle.

It's like trying to get rid of a habit with effort. What you will get is strengthening the habit instead of weakening it. To change it, simply create a new image of yourself where this habit no longer exists. After that, it doesn't matter whether you insist on doing it or avoiding it. The mental image, if kept alive and made real for the mind, cannot help but find expression in reality through thoughts, emotions and actions. It's Law! Just as an acorn manifests the essence / image / information of the oak contained in its core, you manifest yourself.

And now let's move on to the practical phase, so how to cure the inferiority complex?

First, identify in which situations in your life you feel this feeling of inferiority arising. Once identified, mentally create a new image of yourself as you go through these situations. Feel comfortable in these situations. Now you are relaxed, you have everything under control, there is nothing wrong, you do not feel inferior to anyone. The better mental image of you that you have created must be able to arouse emotions in you but if you still do not feel anything do not worry. The important thing at the moment is that you are clear about where you want to go. Now, to reach that emotional place , as mentioned before, we need to relax ...

Lie down or sit in an armchair, relax all the muscles, let go. Consciously release all muscle tension. And now, to sink completely into this relaxation, mentally imagine your body as if it were that of a puppet. Hands, wrists, arms, legs ... the joints no longer exist and everything is held together by threads. Mentally loosen all these threads. Your body is now lying without any tension, it is unable to move.

When you feel you have reached a good state of relaxation, recall the mental image of yourself that you created earlier, in this way you will strengthen it.

This exercise if repeated daily will bring you enormous benefits. Of course you can use it for other purposes as well as to overcome the inferiority complex.

Simply relaxing from the accumulated tensions very often is already enough to untie the mental and emotional knots that we have naively created. On the contrary, fighting something with the simple effort of the will does nothing but generate more tension, therefore it allows the persistence of the situation we want to dissolve.

THE EQUATION THAT CREATES REALITY

And to conclude I would like to remind you of the importance of mental images. This is the equation that allows us to experience life:

IMAGE + SOUND = EMOTION

Emotion is what makes you feel alive, why? Because emotion is the only thing that is truly real, or rather, it is the only thing that can deceive (deceive) your mind and make it believe that the associated image is true. The mind experiences reality (image + sounds) that you offer it in a more or less intense way based on the volume of the emotion you associate with it. Notice, all the memories you have are more or less vivid based on the emotions you felt in those moments. If you didn't feel emotions now you wouldn't remember anything. The emotion allows the writing and overwriting of the unconscious .

That's why just wanting isn't enough. If you want more you have to be grateful! If imagining a better life fails to arouse emotion in the long run, you won't even be able to imagine it anymore because the image loses its nourishment. Conversely, if the image of the best life you desire manages to arouse strong emotions of anticipated enthusiasm and gratitude in you, you can be sure that something in your unconscious has set in motion and from now on you will be guided towards that image. with the aim of concretizing it on the physical plane. And I'm sorry if I repeat myself but I will never tire of telling you: What you already feel yours is what you will have. What you think you are you will be!

Forget the inferiority complex, you are a unique and unrepeatable being. And you know what? The only reason you are here is to project as much light as possible, to create wonder. So, first of all, relax... and then shine!

Conclusion

To start training the mind and balancing the hemispheres as announced before, there are specific exercises that allow the athlete to get into the ring calm, serene and confident of their abilities to the point of marveling at being free of agitation before the match.

In the state of Flow we do not think about the future, nor about the past, but we only live the PRESENT in full confidence of our own means and potential.

There is no doubt of making mistakes, there are no limiting thoughts, no internal dialogue, but everything is FLUID!

Those who think and do not act end up being depressed. Whoever acts without thinking risks madness. Only the thought of a disciplined mind followed by disciplined action can bring you those changes you desire. Thinking is easy, acting is difficult, and putting your thoughts into practice is the hardest thing in the world!